The Physician's Nutritionist

My Secret to Permanent Weight Loss

To June —
You Can do this —
All The Best —
Freddy K.

by
Freddy Kaye, PhD, L.D.

**Thirty Years of Counseling Overweight and Obese People as
PhD Clinical Nutritionist and Licensed Dietitian**

MW00973320

© 2014 Freddy Kaye, Ph.D, L.D.
DrFreddyKaye@yahoo.com (email)
www.ThePhysiciansNutritionist.com (website)
All Rights Reserved.

No part of this book may be reproduced, stored in a retrieval system,
or transmitted by any means without the written permission of the author.
ISBN: 978-1-4259-2766-0

Printed in the United States of America
Tallahassee, Florida

This book is printed on 30% Post-Consumer Recycled Paper.

Book Design by CuneoCreative.com, Tallahassee, Florida
Cover and back cover photos by Mark Wallheiser

Table of Contents

Acknowledgements

This book is the written result of 30-plus years of counseling thousands of individuals, couples and families for an overwhelming life problem. However, it could not have been completed without major "help from my friends" who are, for the most part, my dear relatives as well.

I would very much like to thank my lovely wife, Susan, both for putting up with me in general AND for editing this book. She is a woman of great patience and intelligence *(yet many of my close friends question her intelligence because she is married to me!)*.

Next, my daughter, Lily, PhD, Counseling Psychology *(with a research specialty in Health Psychology)* from the University of Florida and also my other editor.

Also, my friend Mark Riley, PhD, Quantum Physicist at FSU who was persistent in keeping after me to do this.

I very much thank them for their support because they knew how important this work is to me. I have a message which needs to be proclaimed to those who need to hear it.

Introduction

What gives me the right to call myself The Physician's Nutritionist? Good question!

During the past seven years, a series of physicians have come to my office to lose weight. This includes a variety of different kinds of doctors: pulmonologist, orthopedic surgeon, pediatrician, OB/GYN, family practice physicians...

Why would they do this when they already have medical knowledge about obesity, you might ask?

Well, because losing weight is complex and multi-faceted. It requires much more than medical knowledge alone. Losing weight is about behavior shaping, lifestyle change, habit forming, learning about and challenging yourself, and most importantly, developing an approach that is sustainable.

We all know the phrase "Eat Less, Exercise More." Okay, great, thanks. Not particularly helpful.

That is clearly not enough to help you make realistic lifestyle changes, accomplish permanent weight loss, and obtain the level of health you probably desire.

Of all people, physicians know so much about how the body works on a biological and chemical level. Realistically, though, that knowledge is often not enough at the moment you pick up a menu and decide what to order. So many other factors are at play...psychology, motivation, social influence, environment...

In addition to having helped physicians successfully lose weight, I also refer to myself as the Physician's Nutritionist because (a) I have trained many young health professionals on the treatment of obesity and related health problems, and (b) physicians often send their patients to me for diet- or obesity-related health problems, none of which can be solved with a prescription or a few minutes of advice.

For the past 25 years, I have been on the faculty of the Family Practice Residency program of Tallahassee Memorial Hospital, which partners with Florida State University's medical school and other programs. My role has been teaching young family practice physicians how to help their patients with both weight and weight- or diet-related problems such as Type II diabetes, high blood pressure, high cholesterol/elevated lipids, IBS *(irritable bowel syndrome)*, and gastroesophageal reflux.

Through working with a wide variety of people, from a wide variety of backgrounds, over multiple decades, I have learned the "Secret" to Permanent Weight Loss.

What is the Secret? The Secret to Permanent Weight Loss is establishing a specific kind of ROUTINE – or structure and consistency – of what, when, and how much you eat. The Secret is engaging in specific behaviors at a frequency that actually TRAINS your body to work differently. With the right types of foods, portions, and timing, as well as incorporating fat-burning exercise *(Power Walking!)* into your lifestyle, you can TEACH YOUR BODY TO LET GO of the excess fat that it is holding on to.

The approach of the Physician's Nutritionist is realistic, flexible/personalizable and effective!

I know that you can do it because I have seen this approach work for not only so MANY people, but also all different kinds of people. Whether you are doctor or patient, Generation Y or baby boomer, I can direct you on your journey to stop struggling with the most expensive and most frustrating medical problems we face today...overweight and obesity. Weight no more. Let's go!

Most Sincerely,

Freddy Kaye, PhD, L.D.
Clinical Nutritionist and
Expert at Helping People
Lose Weight permanently

The Physicians

I have been very pleased with my relationship with Freddy Kaye. He has empowered me to lose weight and improve my overall health by teaching me a new way of approaching eating and exercise. His method is not a "diet" as we typically think of in American culture in that I am not counting calories or "points" and I am not avoiding foods that I enjoy. He has taught me how to plan my nutritional intake to meet my needs without really sacrificing any of the foods that I LOVE TO EAT! He has also helped me to identify and mitigate the effect of stressors that trigger some of my bad food choices. His plan for me has been practical in that it has been easy to incorporate into the eating patterns of my large family and I have been able to eat in restaurants frequently while still having success in my overall program. He has been patient with me as I have had some stumbles on my road to success. I truly believe that I now have the tools needed to control my weight and health long term. I also believe that I would have failed in my quest to achieve control of my weight and health if I had not had Freddy's guidance.

John S. Thabes, MD
Pulmonologist

My name is Lorene D. Ligouri, MD and I am now retired from a very busy practice of Obstetrics and Gynecology. I left Brooklyn, NY and retired here. During many of my years in active practice, I had the honor of being listed in a consumer guide published by Castle and Conley, known as: The Best Doctors of the New York Metro Area. With this "wealth" of experience and fund of knowledge, it is now my great pleasure to recommend Dr. Freddy Kaye for all your nutritional needs. Many years ago, a young woman in my practice, required a referral and added, "send me to someone that you would send a relative to; someone that you would send your mother or your sister to". Since then, I have thought about this young woman many times. Dr. Kaye is the physician that I would send my loved ones to. Dr. Kaye is knowledgeable and gives lectures to large medical groups; he teaches resident physicians at Tallahassee Memorial Hospital and is able to stay up to date on nutritional topics that are forever changing.

I am one of those individuals who has been overweight "almost since birth". Weight Watchers must have a permanent folder for me, even though the weight loss has never been permanent. Dr. Kaye has actually been able to provide me with sensible menu planning. As a result, I have lost 35 lbs and have been able to keep this weight off for over 3 years. His medical background makes him the nutritionist most ideally suited to take care of other doctors, difficult patients or those who represent "a challenge". Dr Kaye has helped me with weight loss. Even more important, he has helped me to cope with the dietary consequences of illness. I am 60 years old now and have multiple, complicated, medical conditions. Dr. Kaye has always been there for me. It is without reservation that I am now able to support Dr. Kaye's diet and his most recent book.

Lorene D. Ligouri, MD, OBGYN

I met Dr Freddy Kaye when I was a resident at the Tallahassee Memorial Family Practice Residency Program over 20 years ago. He was my teacher then and a strong promoter of good nutrition and regular exercise. He is still pushing the same message with different caveats and local choices. Over the years our paths have crossed multiple times and I have found him to be as true a person in or out of the office. He is genuine and cares about what he teaches. He not only talks the walk, he preaches it and walks it as well.

As time has dealt its cruel blow to me with gravity as its henchman, I have sought his services and advice on a regular basis. He has commonsense approaches to everyday habits dealing with eating and weight management with proper nutrition and exercise.

He is knowledgeable about ethnic foods from different cultures as he has lived in European and Caribbean areas for long periods of time. With this depth of cultural experiences, he is uniquely adapted and culturally sensitive to the needs of varied races of people

David A. Keen MD, MPH
Family Practice

"Dr. Kaye's system of weight loss and maintenance is straight-forward and very easy to follow. I use it myself. Unlike many of the popular fad diets, Dr. Kaye emphasizes lifestyle change and a balanced diet that does not leave out any essential nutrients. He "sweetens the pot" with concrete tips to help you be successful, many of which I, a physician, had never heard before I worked with him. His system can be followed successfully for years. I have witnessed this in many of his clients. In a world in which 90% of those who lose weight gain it back within a year, this is a very positive statement. I strongly recommend this program. It is culturally sensitive to the needs of varied races of people"

D. Paul Robinson, MD, F.A.A.P.
Pediatrics

Dr. Freddy Kaye provides a basic, no-nonsense plan to weight loss. Stressing routine, not gimmicks, he coaches you along your journey with helpful hints and strategies. More importantly, his overall apporach is toward the goal of healthier living and weight maintenance. I have seen first-hand many of his "successes" who are now happier, healthier and lighter…"

Floyd Jaggears, MD
Orthopedic Surgeon

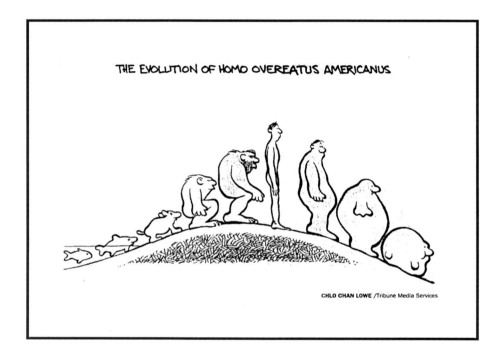

Why This Book and Why This Author?

Losing weight and keeping it off is difficult. Many see it as impossible. But after over two and a half decades of successful nutrition counseling, I have found the secrets, and I'm going to share them with you.

Otherwise, why buy this book? I mean, who wants or needs another diet book or weight loss book? Perhaps, dear reader, you do.

I am asking you to come with me on a journey. Not through the Twilight Zone, but on a path to a slimmer, healthier you. Begin by doing what I suggest for one month...for one lousy, 'stinkin' month. If you do, you will see results, I promise. The key is to focus on thinking before you eat. You will begin the process of consciously changing your eating habits, changing your awareness, your attitude and above all – your lifestyle. And, you will begin to feel great.

Making healthy food choices and increasing your metabolism are important, but changing the habits and behaviors that have caused you to gain the weight in the first place will help you to lose weight permanently. There is one behavior in particular that can make a tremendous difference. Wait, what are you thinking? Exercise? Diet? Muzzle? *(Just kidding)* No.

The behavior is... ROUTINE, routine and consistency. This sounds simple, yet many people find it difficult to accomplish.

But with routine you can turn your body into a well oiled, efficient machine.

Let's begin on this path. How did you get to where you are today? Where did those pounds actually come from? The problem, at least half of you might say, is your "slowing metabolism." What would you say if I asked you about your metabolism? "Mine has stopped!" "Mine left me 10 years ago!" "Mine took the last flight to Terra Del Fuego!" "What metabolism? I'm pretty sure I don't have one!"

Yes, your metabolism, the rate you burn off calories, does slow down as you grow older. At 25 years old, your metabolism automatically decreases by eight percent, and it continues to slow down eight percent every 10 years. That's the bad news. More bad news is that with poor nutritional habits, this slowing could start to happen at any age. You could blame it on your parents and say you genetically inherited a slow metabolism. However, what's more likely is that your parents just didn't know enough about nutrition or metabolism to teach you what you needed to know.

It is time to get over that. Instead of blaming your parents, which is always a wonderfully opportunistic thing to do, you must realize that the art of parental nutrition teaching did not exist. All parents can agree – there was no Parenthood 101 book handed to you – and even if there had been, "Child Nutrition" probably would not have been the first chapter you turned to. I mean, who knew?

One of my favorite authors, Dr. Scott Peck, wrote a book in 1978 titled "The Road Less Traveled." It has sold over six million copies in North America alone and has been translated into over 20 different languages. On the first page of the book is the following sentence: "Life is difficult."

You and I may likely reply, "No Kidding!" or as any teenager might say "Duh! Get a Grip!" The truth is that your slowing metabolism is not the main culprit here. Think about it: not all "older people" are overweight, right? We cannot just blame it on your parents or your genetics and be done with it. Life is more complicated than that and so is weight control. An inconsistent lifestyle and bad habits are what got you where you are today.

But no worries...because I am here as your guide and your coach, ready to educate you on how to lose weight permanently! You dig? I have been professionally counseling people who are overweight and obese for more than 30 years. I see 15-18 people daily, five days a week. My clients range from being 15 pounds overweight *(looking at them, you might say, "Where, in your right eyelid?")* to 300 pounds overweight *(yes, 300 pounds overweight)*. My largest client weighed 516 pounds. Many of my clients weigh 300 to 350 pounds. Another client was a 7 year old boy who weighed 206 pounds...He was accompanied by his 424 pound mom! To quote her: "We come from a long line of big people." Fifteen percent of my clients in private practice are children. A few have specific eating disorders such as bulimia or binge eating disorder.

I am a teacher and a counselor. For 25 years, I have also been teaching diet therapy to young physicians at a highly regarded Family Practice Residency Program, so that they can have a better understanding of weight control and diet-related diseases. I also have taught a required nutrition class to nursing and pharmacology students at Florida A&M University *(FAMU)*.

I have a Masters of Science degree in Nutrition and Food Science and a PhD in Adult Education with a specialization in Nutrition Education. Both degrees are from Florida State University *(FSU)*. For a complete biography, please look to the final page of this book.

Although I have spent many years in school, my real education has come from my one-on-one and small group counseling. I have found that the most common thread that affects all people who battle their weight is the lack of a routine, and that the best way to combat this lack of a routine is by giving them a path to follow.

I am going to explain the process, give examples of the problem, and help you to understand that no one is perfect and that failure can be just momentary. Remember this childhood lesson: "Pick yourself up, dust yourself off, and start all over again." It can come in handy in more scenarios than just a spill off the old tricycle.

My Personal Overweight History

If you saw me now, 5'9" and 165 pounds, you might wonder, "What the heck does this guy know about being overweight?" In fact, I know quite a lot. When I graduated from high school, I weighed 155 pounds. During college at Tulane University, I lifted weights, drank beer, ate burgers, and went up to 180 pounds - some muscle, some fat, but I was "strong like bull."

During college, tragedy struck my family. Both of my parents died unexpectedly. After college, I attempted law school back home in Miami. I was a psychological wreck. My head and neck *(both growing)* were united by pizza. I went to the "white psychologist," also known as the refrigerator, for my emotional strokes. It provided a temporary therapy that did nothing but make me feel worse later on.

I quit law school after a year and moved to California, then tipping the scales at 192 pounds. Fortunately for me, the neighbors in the apartment above me were slim and health-conscious and they liked telling me why! I hated them. Plus, this one skinny guy had two skinny girlfriends *(what?!)*. Boy, did I hate him!

I learned that these neighbors did not eat much meat, and they routinely walked most places. They were fit, trim and happy. I, on the other hand, was desperate. My clothes did not fit, and I hated the way I looked. My self-esteem was non-existent, and I was ready to try anything.

So, for six months, I began to eat less meat. I ate starches primarily and walked almost daily. At the end of those six months, I had lost 40 pounds and felt great. Most importantly, I had learned how to lose weight properly, my first shot at it. I was hooked on nutrition and on changing my lifestyle. It was 1968, the perfect time for change! I was changing my awareness of what I should eat and my attitude was focused on what I really wanted for myself. I decided I wanted to look good, feel good, have energy, and have confidence in myself — and, it happened. Eureka!!!

With this new-found discovery, I began to read, learn, and ponder questions such as: Where does fat really come from in our diet? Why do so many people die from heart attacks and strokes? Why do so many people have type 2 diabetes? Why do so many people have cancer? And, for goodness sake, why are there so many obese people in America? *(That was in 1968 and look at us now! Yikes!)* Things have definitely gotten worse. Over 66 percent of adults in America are now overweight or obese![1] Astounding!

Some Basic Facts Regarding Obesity That We Should All Know

- Obesity increases the risk of illness for approximately 30 serious medical conditions.
- Obesity is associated with increases in death from all causes.
- An earlier onset of obesity-related diseases, such as type 2 diabetes, is occurring among children and adolescents with obesity.
- Individuals with obesity are at higher risk for impaired mobility.
- Overweight or obese individuals experience social stigmatization and discrimination in employment and academic situations.

Still, it took some time for me to realize that I wanted to be part of the solution. For six years, I lived and worked in Copenhagen, London, and Paris, yet my mind continued to focus on nutrition and the health problems that people in America were having because of their inadequate knowledge of how to eat healthy and have a healthy lifestyle. I decided to answer my calling and go back to school. In 1975, I moved from Paris, France, to Tallahassee, Florida *(just a little bit different)*, and entered Florida State University to begin my quest to educate people on how to take better care of themselves. Now, I sometimes joke to myself about my choice to become a Clinical Nutritionist. If I had known how difficult it would be to get people to change their lifestyles, I might have become a plumber instead! (*"Lady, the faucet is leaking. That'll be fifty bucks. Do you want me to fix it? Yes or no? There's nothing in between!"*) But nobody warned me.

So, here I am today, transferring my experience from working with thousands of clients on how to live a healthier lifestyle and how to lose weight into a succinct guide for others who are trying to do the same. This is not a diet book on how you should restrict your life. Instead, it is a guide for living in such a way that your life won't be restricted - by your body or by your health.

The Protein Fast

Long before there was the Atkins Diet *(yes, there was life before Atkins)*, there was another high protein, no carbohydrate diet, the Stillman Diet, which originated in the early 1950s because as America's food availability grew, so did our waistlines. People who want to lose weight quickly *regardless* of health concerns or longevity of their weight loss success should be grateful for Atkins.

On the plus side, people on the Atkins diet lose *(water)* weight quickly and thus become motivated. Depending primarily on protein *(meat, poultry, fish, dairy products and eggs)* for energy and not receiving any carbohydrates *(starches)*, the body begins to burn fat for fuel, resulting in dramatic weight loss. And you're hooked! Your cholesterol production may even decrease. Even more to be hooked about!

But potentially serious problems are ahead. Over time, too much protein can lead to kidney failure, because the kidneys have to filter the end products of protein - urea, uric acid and ammonia. At increased levels, they are dangerous poisons for the body. Too much protein also causes gout and kidney stones with painful symptoms.

The type of protein you choose also makes a difference. Many people on Atkins or similar diets choose protein from sources that are high in fat and high in saturated fat, such as red meat and whole milk dairy products. These fats tend to combine with the cholesterol your cells produce to form plaque, which can block your arteries. This can lead to heart disease, especially because you may not know the plaque is building up until major problems arise.

Want to hear more? While you are on the Atkins Diet you are not changing the habits and behaviors that caused the weight gain in the first place. You are just backing off CARBS, eating more protein, and "La De Da, I'm doing great." Not so! If you don't change the habits and behaviors that caused you to gain weight, you'll just end up in the weight gain, weight loss, weight gain never-ending cycle.

Another thing to consider: there is no FIBER in meat, dairy or eggs. The usual cause of chronic constipation is not consuming enough dietary fiber. Ingested insoluble fiber helps clean your intestines by keeping foods continuously moving through the colon and reducing the time that cancer-causing substances remain in the digestive tract, thus helping to prevent cancer of the colon. Soluble fiber is important because it delays the emptying of food from the stomach, resulting in a more uniform absorption of carbohydrates and improving glucose control. It also aids in cholesterol elimination.

Getting On The
The Physician's
Nutritionist Program

Let's get started. Recall, I am asking you to take a month, one lousy month, to please do what I suggest. One month - no excuses - just do it.

First, I want you to look at the habits and the behaviors that have caused you to gain the weight in the first place. Without doing that, you will not change those behaviors, no matter what over-zealous diet you may have been on. A "diet" suggests temporarily following someone else's formula. Instead, I am asking you to go down a path, armed with knowledge, toward a healthy future.

I marvel at both the amount of money and the human effort being spent annually on weight loss programs: 30 billion dollars a year! What an incredible waste of energy and resources, especially when the solution is so simple. Look at the cause of the problem, change it, go down this path, create the right habits, and you're there! So now, onto the program...

What is the program? The program is the weight loss journey I am asking you to go on. While you are on this path, you will do great...you will do great the majority of the time, but occasionally you will "blow it" by wandering off the program *(we all do)*. It is not a question of if, but of when. So what happens when you do blow it or fall off program and lose your way? What happens is this: the next meal, the next day, you get right back on the program. This is not about all or nothing. Nobody is perfect here. If you blow it, just get right back on it, OK? OK!

Needs vs. Wants

Often, you wait too long to eat. You are working on a project at the office, it is 1 p.m., and hunger sets in. You are starving. As usual, you probably haven't eaten breakfast, and now you are more than ready for lunch. What do you want? "Glad you asked! Today I'm craving a Big Mac, medium fries and a medium coke. Yes, a real coke...none of that diet stuff!" So you go to the drive-thru and get what you want - along with 1,130 calories, mucho grams of fat *(29 grams in the Big Mac alone)* and plenty of guilt *(Jewish guilt, Catholic guilt, your mother's guilt, it's all the same)*. And you blow it. And then you think, "What the heck, I've already blown it for the day, make it a 16oz. vanilla milkshake!" *(Add 550 calories and 13 grams of fat.)* So you keep blowing it, and the rest is history.

Ask yourself, "WHAT DO I REALLY WANT?" Well, easy answer. "I want to feel good, look good, wear certain clothes, be healthy and finally be in control of my weight. That's what I want!" So if you get what you *need*, food-wise, you will *then* get what you really want. You dig? Yes!

The Balance in Life

If I had spent 10 years in a dark but enlightening cave, I might take a stab at telling you the meaning of life. I can't do that, but as a person who has lost weight and kept it off for the past 45 years, I can tell you the secrets of weight loss.

Too often, I meet clients who are workaholics or very involved parents. They do everything for everyone else and put themselves "DFL," Dead Finally Last. That's the wrong way to go. Wrong!

An example: You're a mom with two school-aged children. Dad thinks he is so important that he must get to his job first. So he is gone, and you're left to clothe, feed, and deliver two children to school or the bus stop. Then, it is time for you to go to work. Your boss asks you to work through lunch to get a last-minute report out. In the interest of time, you grab a quickie fried chicken sandwich. At the end of the day, you rush to pick-up the children from after-school care because your husband has an unforeseen meeting. Then, you head for home. On the way, the children are hungry and whiny, and you can barely take it. As soon as you get home, everyone races to the kitchen for a pre-dinner snack. You stand at the kitchen counter, anesthetizing your brain and stomach with high-caloric comfort. Stop. Tell me what's wrong with this picture? There is no balance in your life, and you are too harried to be a nutritional example for your children.

BALANCE must include taking equal time for you. In order to take care of others, you need to take care of yourself first. The above example could have just as easily been the other partner in the relationship. Dad could be experiencing the same situation. Being out of balance relates to us all.

I have just given you an example of a life without balance. What does a life with balance look like? A life with balance means making/taking the time to eat right, exercise and de-stress. You can do it. There are ways to bring balance into your life.

For example: To exercise, get up earlier in the morning before everyone else needs to get ready for school or work. Take a brisk 30 minute walk. Another idea: if you have an hour for lunch, spend half of it walking and half of it eating *(you will have more time if you bring a healthy lunch from home or a frozen meal)*. Or, leave work at a specific time and exercise before you go home. If you're a workaholic, you are less likely to leave work on time to go exercise and NOBODY is going to tell you, "Hey, stop working! Enough already! Go to the gym or go walk, get out of here!" There's probably no one to tell you anyway because everyone else has already left! Are you starting to get the picture? As we get more into behaviors, I will further elaborate on how to create time in your daily life that will allow you to have the balance needed to walk forward down this path.

Diet Misconceptions, Misinformation, Missed the Boat

There is so much diet misinformation out there. Who to believe? What is the truth? What are carbohydrates, the good, the bad, and the simple or complex? Are starches fattening? Should I never eat bread again? Does Atkins really work and why or why not? Is Sugar Busters the way to go? How about the Grapefruit Diet? *(I mean, have you ever met a fat grapefruit? Pleasingly plump maybe, but not fat!)* Is there anyone who can tell me the truth about all this nonsense?

Thankfully, you are in luck! I will begin with carbohydrates. Many people are confused about the differences between simple and complex carbohydrates. Others do not know that there are actually different kinds of carbohydrates. Carbohydrates are one of three macronutrients in our diets that provide calories. The other two are protein and fat. Carbohydrates provide most of the energy needs in our daily lives for normal body functions and for exercise. Carbohydrates are considered either simple or complex, based on their chemical structure. Both types contain 4 calories per gram. Both are also digested into a blood sugar called glucose, which is then used to fuel our bodies for work or exercise. Simple carbohydrates or the commonly termed "bad carbs" are digested quickly. Many simple carbohydrates contain

refined sugars and few or no vitamins and minerals. Examples
include: fruit juice, candy, honey, molasses, sugar, baked goods
made with white/refined flour *(including white bread, white pastas,
etc.)*, and regular sodas.

Complex carbohydrates or "good carbs" take longer to digest
and are usually packed with fiber, vitamins and minerals.
Examples are: whole wheat breads, whole grain cereals and
pastas, beans, peas, lentils, and brown rice. Complex
carbohydrates are starches and NOT fattening **unless you eat too
much of them!** When you eat brown rice, whole grain noodles,
sweet potatoes, whole grain cereals and bread, couscous, beans,
peas *(but not green English peas)* and lentils, for example, they will
SLOWLY be converted into sugar and stored in your liver as
glycogen or "stored sugar." Since your body needs sugar for
energy *(breathing, talking, walking, whatever)*, the liver slowly
releases it into your bloodstream, almost like a time-released
capsule. In about four hours, your liver uses up its stored energy
and is ready to be re-fed. Starch, in and of itself, is never
fattening. All beans – such as kidney beans, butter beans, black
beans, red beans, garbanzo beans *(chick peas)*, and navy beans,
whether they are canned, frozen, fresh or dried – are starches.
Peas – such as black-eyed peas, white-acre peas *(straight from the
Ol' South)*, pigeon peas *(from the Caribbean and Africa)*, chick peas
(from the Mediterranean), or lentils *(from India)* – are also starches.
Eight ounces of peas or beans have only 200 calories and give
you sustained energy and much-needed fiber, plus they taste
good with the right low-fat seasoning.

So starches are not fattening, unless you eat too much of them!
If you have ever thought to yourself, "Wow, that potato was
really good. I'll have another!" Whoa, wait a sec, now we have a
problem! Your liver is going to say to the next baked potato,
"Excuse me second potato, we have no more room for you in

here. You will have to go around the corner to talk to Mr. FAT about storage! See you later!" This is why and how starch becomes fattening. That is a pretty easy image to picture, huh? Also, when our bodies run out of room for fat, they create more fat cells to store it. Who needs more fat cells, I ask you?

Fat Cells (Ugh!)

Did you lose any sleep last night wondering how some people could weigh 489 pounds or even more? You didn't? Well, I've seen it, and now I am going to tell you, so you'll know!

How does one become an extremely overweight or obese adult? There are normally two periods in a young child's life when FAT CELLS can be created: 0-2 years old and 7-12 years old. But it doesn't necessarily stop there. Even adults can create more FAT CELLS.

Here's what happens: At eight months old, little Johnny is being bottle-fed. After a while, his body sends a message to his brain, telling him that it satisfied. So, while Dad is feeding him the bottle, little Johnny turns his head or pushes the bottle away. He has had enough. But parents, in all their wisdom, believe they need to coax Johnny to finish the bottle "for Dad". *(They never had Parenting 101 in school.)* So, even though he was satisfied and really didn't want any more, little Johnny finishes that last bit of food that his body really didn't want. Now, his body needs to put it somewhere. But where, you ask? "Aha," the body says, "Let's store it; save it just in case! Let's create some new FAT CELLS."

The same situation occurs with 7 year old little Sarah. Mom has given her a great plate of tasty food. Sarah eats for a while and then stops. So Mom coaxes little Sarah, "Come on, honey, finish your food. Clean your plate, and *(guess what folks)* I'll give you ice cream for dessert!" Well, we know even though little

Sarah has had enough, she's no fool...so she cleans her plate *(and now belongs to that age-old American club, the "Clean Plate Club")*. She gets the reward *(dessert)* and has eaten too much. So, "What's a body to do?" Little Sarah's body now creates and stores the extra food in those dreaded *(you guessed it!)* FAT CELLS! Curses!

Now, here's the worst part: Once you have those fat cells, you've got them, and you can never get rid of them. You can reduce the size of the fat cells, but not the quantity. That's why we have plenty of "rather large" people in America. Once you have the fat cells, the body can grow, shrink, and grow some more, but never totally get rid of them.

Do you remember the old admonition: "You better eat the rest of that liver, son *(daughter)*. Think of the starving kids in _____ (fill in the blank for country of starving people) who would also love to have that broccoli."

I have a *(rather morbid but interesting)* theory: You can accurately tell how old someone is by what country the kids were starving in. For example, if you are a baby boomer, then the kids were probably starving in China. Am I right? For my children's generation, it was Somalia... Think about it.

What Is Success?

People often ask me about my "success rate." For years, we all have thought that "success" means reaching your "goal weight." Your goal weight is the magic number that we often pull out of thin air and wish to stay at. Keeping off all the weight you needed to lose is the ideal. Yet, I have realized that success comes in many forms or levels.

The following are all different forms of success:
1. Reaching your goal weight and maintaining it.
2. Losing half of what you need to lose and keeping that off.

19

3. Losing some weight and additionally, lowering your blood pressure and/or blood sugar and reducing the need for/lowering your dosage of various medications.
4. Losing some weight and feeling better because you have more energy, more self-satisfaction, and are more agile. Through making healthier and wiser food choices, you also have better self-esteem and a more positive attitude about your body and your health.
5. Exercising more, walking regularly. Your clothes are looser, and you feel in-control.
6. Not gaining more weight. This is important. Many of us fail to recognize this concept. How many of us continue to gain weight over the years? Where does it stop? How do you stop it? Forget about weight loss for just a moment. What about not gaining?

Some years ago, I had a client in his 40's who weighed 340 pounds. I tried counseling him for two years without success. Now, I really do succeed with a lot of people, otherwise I would not have been able to keep up a busy private practice for 26 years! Finally during one session I told him, "Look, I really am not helping you. You haven't lost any weight." He came in every two weeks, we directed, evaluated, and we made new plans to help him succeed in his journey of weight loss. "We have not had good results. Maybe you should consider seeking counsel elsewhere?"

He looked at me with great surprise and replied, "Are you kidding? You don't understand. I have been everywhere...been counseled by many...and I kept on gaining weight...You ARE helping me...I am not 400 pounds!"

His concept of success was that after many years of continuously gaining, he was finally able to maintain his weight.

He felt he was doing great and succeeding and knew where he would have been if he had never come to see me. That comment opened my eyes.

One aspect that is common to all of these kinds of successes is that success tends to breed success. Once you experience success, you are more likely to either continue being successful or become even more successful. You must think about your definition of success in terms of your own weight loss. You should have a short-term success definition *(goal)* and a long-term success definition *(goal)*. By allowing yourself to experience success and feel proud of yourself, you will be more likely to have the confidence and the motivation to continue further and to reach even higher levels of success. Allow yourself to be successful.

Attention Baby Boomers:

"You talkin' to me?" OK, how do you know you are a Baby Boomer? Well, if you know the words to at least one song of the musical *Hair*. If those mop-haired guys from England became a favorite, possibly most favorite, singing group, I believe they may have been known as *The Beatles*! Again, if you watched *Starsky and Hutch* on TV or possibly *St. Elsewhere*, then you are ...oh wait, today if you are on 6 different medications: Lisinopril for High Blood Pressure, Metformin for Diabetes, Crestor for Elevated Cholesterol, maybe Prosac for Depression, your knees are hurting, your feet, your hips *(we won't even discuss you sex life... "whatever")* You need this book, The Physician's Nutritionist, you need this Program because it takes one to know one! If today you are somewhere close to or between the ages of 58-64 you want to not suffer as you are, not feel badly about your weight as you do now. You want to finally know HOW to lose weight AND finally keep it off... because time and patience is running out... we need to do this "thing" *(Weight Loss)* NOW!

The Philosophy

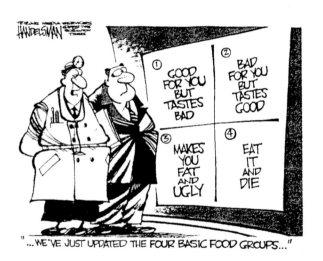

(Handelsman/Tribune Media Services)

Routine, Routine, Routine

OK gang, this is why you are here. This is going to change your life for the better, forever. No kidding! We have gone over the major components of *The Path*, now for the "glue that ties it all together." It is necessary for all the other components and suggestions to work effectively.

Instead of "losing 30 pounds by Friday at noon," you can lose weight and keep it off for life by creating a ROUTINE.

Nearly every weight loss client has had a common thread or a similarity. No matter if they had 20 pounds to lose or 200 pounds, they did not have a routine as to when they ate, how much they ate, and even what they ate. Trust me on this. *(I know when someone says, "Trust me", you may think "run", but not now.)* In some ways, this is so simple and yet many people find it quite difficult to accomplish.

IF YOU EAT *(approximately)* THE SAME AMOUNT OF CALORIES, AT THE SAME TIME EACH DAY, AND THE SAME AMOUNT OF FOOD, your body says to itself, "I know I'm going to be taking in calories, so I'll give off some calories." But when you have no routine in your eating behaviors, your body gets confused. Let's say that on most mornings you skip breakfast, and then one morning you decide to eat breakfast. Since you eat breakfast, you wait later than usual to eat lunch, so then you are hungry and you eat more lunch than usual. So now your body is very confused, and now it doesn't trust you. *(Aha!)* After some deliberation, the body decides that the best idea is to save or store

23

whatever calories it receives, because it really does not know when and how much it will be fed next. Herein lies the problem.

One past client weighed 435 pounds when she came into my office for the first time. She reported that she ate one meal a day - supper *(I wondered if supper typically lasted from 6 p.m. to 10 p.m....just kidding...bad joke)*. She rarely ate breakfast or lunch. Only eating one meal per day, she simply could not understand why she was so big and why she could not lose weight.

Another client I had would not eat breakfast *(pretty typical in our society)*. She would get ready quickly and rush off to work in the morning. By 10 a.m., the coffee and doughnuts would be calling her name, "Hey Jennifer, we're over here!" She would then eat a couple of doughnuts and by 11:30 a.m., be ravenous. Her blood sugar had dropped, hunger had set in, and her lunch plan was non-existent. When her co-workers decided to make a quick trip to McDonald's to bring back a burger, fries and large coke, she said, "Me too!"

When what you eat is a knee-jerk reaction, amounts and choices suffer. If I was standing at the "Pearly Gates" and Saint Peter said to me, "In your 30 years of helping people lose weight, what have you found to be the major problem? Why are people baffled that they can not keep their weight off, if and when they lose weight?" I would tell Saint Peter, "Sir, it is one word: Routine." And then, hopefully he would say to me *(hiding his belly under his robe)*, "You know, I've always wondered what that secret was! You may now enter!"

Back on earth, look at your own daily life and seriously ask yourself:

"Do I have routine when it comes to food?"

Maybe your routine is no routine at all. We all have a routine of some sort. You routinely get up in the morning, brush your teeth, etc., get the kids going, push your partner out of bed, trip over the dog and put on some respectable clothes for work. Then, you routinely drive the same route to work. But what is your routine with food? Let's stop and think for a moment. Did you eat breakfast? Did you bring it with you? What will you eat for lunch? Where will you eat lunch? Did you bring an afternoon snack so you don't hit the snack machines down the hall (*I've been spying on you!*)? And, while we are at it, what's for dinner? "Hey, leave me alone. I haven't even eaten breakfast yet..." you are saying. OK, don't get so huffy. I'm just trying to help.

PLANNING + ORGANIZATION = CONTROL

Generally, having a shopping list with breakfast, lunch and supper foods listed is a start. Pardon my simplification, but I am asking you to consider <u>creating a weekly menu</u>...a list of "what do I need to eat for each of these meals?" See the sample menu as a possible guideline to follow.

By planning some meals, grocery shopping will become easier (*it is amazing how many people, particularly single people, do not food shop regularly*). Planning your meals and shopping regularly will enable you to have the right food available at the right time. Yeah! <u>Once you are organized</u> and have thought about what you will eat this week, it <u>is easy to eat the right amount of the right food on a routine basis.</u> Feeling rebellious? Maybe you are thinking, "I always have to have a darn routine with everything! I have a routine with work, school, the kids, my partner, paying bills and working around the house/yard. I'm tired of a routine! I just want to eat when I want to eat, so don't tell me what to do!"

OK, fine then, if you never want to be successful at losing weight and keeping it off, forget about the need for a routine. In fact, go ahead and eat this book! It's high in fiber. No, wait...Do Not Eat This Book! Just give the book to your co-worker who weighs 325 pounds and allow her to read it. She may become a

25

believer and realize how much sense it makes to gain control over her daily life. She could, over the next two years, become a normal weight person and two years after that, still be keeping her weight off. You may be sorry you didn't keep the book

Discipline is a Must in a Weight Loss Battle

We want results NOW. Yesterday would be better. Ok, we'll try to have patience for a little longer, but not much, particularly with weight loss.

Even though it took – who knows how many years – of overindulgence to gain weight, we want it gone now. Many of us who battle our weight problem do not recognize the need to understand weight as a "problem".

As with any problem, we need to learn how to deal with it. There is a method, but we must learn a few premises. The first premise is: <u>You must have discipline</u>.

EASY WEIGHT LOSS IS NOT THE ANSWER!

People who accept the need to change their life find that weight loss becomes much less difficult. Those who try to find easy ways to lose weight rarely succeed.

The answer is DISCIPLINE. "Discipline is the basic key to solving life's problems. Without discipline we can solve nothing," so states Peck, the psychotherapist.

Think about it. How often do we procrastinate because we do not want to experience aggravation or pain? And solving problems, including a weight problem, can be painful. For instance, walking or exercising is an important component to losing weight. However, rising at 6 a.m., a little earlier than usual, is certainly not as pleasant as reading the morning paper while languishing over your freshly brewed cup of java. But despite this, you do decide to take a brisk early walk. This is discipline. *(Plus, these days you could still catch the news through a podcast on your I-pod or by watching it while walking on the treadmill at many gyms!)*

So what is the alternative? Aha! It is to wait until after work. Yet all day long, in the deep recesses of your conniving mind, you must blithely remind yourself of that promise, to walk after work. If you don't look forward to it, it will just be hanging over your head all day, like one more assignment to do.

Some of us just might do it, but most will again put it off until the next day, and then the next. Where is the discipline? As Peck states, "What makes life difficult is that the process of confronting and solving problems is a painful one."

You Don't Achieve Without Sacrifices

There is great value in changing the way you perceive gratification, as in not getting the full-fat ice cream we really, really want but instead, settling for the small cup of low-fat frozen yogurt. Yes, learn to get what you need, not just what you want, because if you do this, you will then get what you really want. You will look good, feel good, like yourself and be in control. The moral of the story: If life is a series of problems, of which your weight is one, discipline and small sacrifices are required.

It may not be easy, but it is manageable. Just do not expect it all tomorrow or the next day, but gradually work to recognize your problems and correct them. Over time, you can succeed at overcoming your problem of being overweight.

Learn to Think Ahead

Where will I be? When will I get there? What food will be available? These are questions you need to ask yourself. People who are successful at permanent weight loss learn to think ahead and analyze a food situation *before* they get knee-deep into it.

For example: It's Saturday morning, 11 a.m., and you are off to the mall to shop and meet some friends. Suddenly, a few hours later, you realize it's now 1 p.m. Hunger hits. Your friend says, "There's Pizza Hut. Let's go eat." By this time, your blood sugar has dropped and emotion has overtaken reason, and you soon find yourself consuming a fat laden, extra cheese pizza. Out of control!!

What if you had done this instead: What if, upon arriving at the mall, you purposely notice where Wendy's *(or another fast food restaurant with one or two healthy choices)* is located and remark to your friends, "Hey, around noon, let's eat there." Now, you have set the stage in your mind and theirs for what your lunch plans will be. So you go off and shop, and then noon hits. You are not feeling hunger pains yet, but you could eat. You tell your friends, "Hey, it's noon, let's stop and go eat." Maybe they reply, "Nah, come on. Let's just go to one more store...then we'll eat." Well, you know going to the next store is unlikely to be a quick trip, so speak up. "Hey, gang, I'm really trying to take care of myself, and I need to eat now, so I'm going over to Wendy's to get a baked potato and a salad. Anybody else want to go now?" You may have some "takers" and maybe not, but if you eat now you'll BEAT THE DROP of your blood sugar and control your appetite by eating and choosing the right food on time. Do this and your body will respond, "Thanks for bringing in those calories that I've been expecting. I'll keep what I need and give off what I don't." And you will be proud of yourself for developing CONTROL! You just did it! Good job! You took control of what you needed to, and it will pay off big time.

Beat the Drop of Your Blood Sugar

This basically means eating before hunger overwhelms you by making better choices, about both amounts and types of food, before you start feeling starved. If you don't, the rest is history.

Feeling great and having lots of energy throughout the day means being able to properly and efficiently metabolize food. More specifically, it involves the break down of sugar into usable energy. The body's ability to regulate levels of sugar in the blood is also important to overall health, weight control, and mood. An effective *(stable)* blood sugar level is the primary source of energy for the body's cells.

When your blood sugar level drops, besides feeling hungry and out of control, you may experience other symptoms like shakiness, headaches, faintness, weakness, dizziness, sweating and even worse. If any of these symptoms occur, you have waited too long to nourish your body *(eat)*. Preventing this from occurring requires getting into a habit of planning where, when and what you will eat. Eventually, it can become automatic. When it does become automatic, on all levels of food planning, then you have created and managed a routine, and you are controlling your weight.

Analyze Your Daily Routine

This doesn't have to be difficult. You just need to think "Where will I be at mealtime?" and "How will I manage my food situation?"

For example: This morning you are going to an office meeting that begins at 11:45 a.m. Sometimes the meeting runs through lunch. As some offices do, they make you wait until the meeting ends to have lunch. Now it is 1:00 p.m., and you're starved. So emotion overtakes reason, and you head to McDonald's. You're thinking, "Cheeseburger, fries and a coke!" Or maybe, the people in charge of the meeting plan more carefully and realize the meeting will last through lunch, so they decide to order out. Of course, their favorite sandwiches and side dishes are pastrami/corned beef with potato salad and chips. So you are a "captive audience," at the mercy of whatever they order, and because that's all there is, you eat it. Wait a minute...you knew that you might be possibly working through lunch. So, PLAN AHEAD. Think to yourself, "OK, I need to nip this situation in the bud!"

Which means you should:

a) Bring a snack such as a cereal bar/granola bar and/or a piece of fruit to stave off hunger until you can get your own lunch *(keep some at the office for those unexpected occurrences)*.

b) Call the person in charge of the meeting and request a turkey/ chicken or lighter sandwich with baked chips if they decide to order lunch in.

c) Make a sandwich at home, and bring it along with a piece of fruit.

d) Bring two healthy sandwiches, and sell the second sandwich for big money to another person in the office who is trying to lose weight! *(Hey, it's just a thought!)*

People get dressed for work in the morning and perhaps even plan what they will wear the night before, yet have no clue as to what they will eat for lunch, let alone supper. Build routine into your life!

My Weight Control/Weight Loss Program

We have discussed some of the concepts involved in weight loss, yet some of you are still asking, "How do I lose 30 pounds by Friday at noon?" Let's take a reality check. You want to lose weight as quickly as possible, of course, but you also want to do it in a reasonable way that is healthy for your body and with behaviors that you will be able to incorporate into your lifestyle for many years down the road. This is an aspect that is not so likely to happen with restrictive, formulaic dieting.

So, what CAN you do? It differs for each person, but <u>it is possible and reasonable to lose 1½ pounds per week - on average - each week</u>. *(That is <u>six pounds per month</u> and <u>72 pounds per year</u>! Not bad, eh?!)* These are pounds that you can not only take off, but keep off.

In order to achieve lasting success, you have to step back and say: "Enough is enough!" Are you ready to seriously look at the habits and behaviors that have caused the weight problems? You must have the attitude that you want to put yourself first, in order to become aware of those habits.

As your guide, your counselor and your coach, I am asking you to get on the program, my program...to really commit yourself to it. While you are on the program, you will do well. When *(not "if")* you "blow it", you must get right back on. Forget the guilt and get right back on. Remember, NOBODY IS

PERFECT. You will blow it at some point, everyone does. But when that happens, instead of moping, you must dust yourself off and get right back on. Part of our difficulties related to staying with a program such as this is our own criteria for success. We tend to have the self-defeating concept of "All or Nothing – I must do it perfectly or not at all." This is not how life works and certainly not how weight loss works. If you are one of the many people out there who judges yourself with this self-defeating concept, you must re-think your definition of success.

An Overview: The Three Main Components

My weight control/weight loss program consists of three major areas of focus. There is more information on each of these three major components in the chapters to follow.

1. Eating the "Ideal Diet"

The first area of focus is the "ideal diet". As children, no one taught us what we should eat or what a portion size is. Our parents didn't really know and there were no guidelines established then. Today, there are specific guidelines from the World Health Organization *(W.H.O.)* as to what really is the "ideal" diet, the diet our bodies were really made to eat. This specific recommendation is a high fiber, complex carbohydrate, low-fat diet with reasonable portions.

2. Increasing Your Metabolism

The second area of focus is increasing your metabolism, which is the rate you burn up calories for energy. To review: The bad news is that your metabolism slows down 8 percent every decade, beginning at the age of 25. An inactive lifestyle will slow your metabolism down even before the age of 25.

But before you close this book in total frustration, there is good news too. You CAN speed up your metabolism. As part of the program, I suggest doing it in three ways:

A) By eating 25 percent of your day's calories at breakfast

B) By being consistent and eating three meals per day, at about the same time each day, and with about the same amount of food per meal

C) By WALKING a minimum of 5 days per week, "speed walking" in the way that I will describe in the chapter on walking

3. Changing Your Habits and Behaviors

The third area of my program focuses on changing the habits and behaviors that caused you to gain the weight in the first place. This will take some serious introspection into your own lifestyle and will require pre-planning, consistency in your behaviors, and establishing routine in your busy life. This subject is discussed throughout the book.

An Overview: The Most Crucial Behavioral Tips

(covered in more detail in the "Changing Your Habits and Behaviors" chapter)

SLOW DOWN YOUR EATING

1. For one week eat supper with the opposite hand from the one you usually use *(if you are right handed use your left hand).*

2. Make a rule: No food on your fork while food is in your mouth.

3. Stop eating in middle of the meal. Put down your fork, and keep your hands in your lap for 1 minute.

SIT DOWN TO EAT *(always)*

✶ **A SPLURGE MEAL ONCE A WEEK**
(Will go into more detail shortly)

WALK
Walk 5-6 days weekly, 30 minutes each day. Water-walking is an alternative for anyone with joint pain, injuries, or other hindrances to walking. *(Or maybe you simply live somewhere where it's "too damn hot.")*

DIET RECALL
Keep your Daily Diet Record. Update your record before each meal. *(Find a template in "The Daily Diet Record and Sample Menu" Chapters).*

PRE-PLAN your menu *(for 5-7 days).* Shop wisely.

BATCH COOK
Batch cook healthy foods regularly over the weekend or on a night that you tend to have a little more time. Then, on days when you don't have time to cook, you will already have healthy options waiting for you in the fridge.

FIRST STEP:
The "Ideal Diet" and Meal Plan Options

Did you seriously lose any sleep last night wondering what your body was *really* made to eat? Wondering what is the perfect, ideal diet? What food choices should we be making for optimum health?

I'm glad you finally asked!

To answer this overwhelming question, we must travel across the world... What do people eat in countries with lower rates of obesity and fewer diet-related diseases? In Japan and China, meals typically include rice and soy products. In India, another one billion plus people, they eat rice, potatoes and peas...and curry. In fact, I've heard that fast food restaurants in India are appropriately called "Curry in a Hurry" *(just kidding)*. Bada ba dum!

Let's move southwestward to Africa. I teach a required class in nutrition for nursing students at a historically Black university, and nearly all of my students are African American. Yet, other students are African and have moved to the U.S. from countries such as Nigeria or Senegal. Each semester, I ask the students who are from Africa to please share with the class what types of foods they typically eat in their home country. The answer *(in the most delightful of accents)* is often something like, "pigeon peas, cassava, yams..." Most of the American students have no real idea of these foods. All of these foods are starches.

In Central and South America, food staples include black

beans, corn and rice. Mexican cuisine uses similar staples but typically with pinto beans instead of black beans. Of course, they also created different types of salsas to make all these starches taste better. *(And good beer to wash this all down, but we won't go there.)*

So, much of the world eats primarily starches. But in America and many other Westernized countries, the dinner plate is based on meat, whether poultry, pork, beef, fish, or something else. We build the whole meal around meat...and then hopefully throw in a starch and something green, to provide color and interest and to fill our plate.

How we conceptualize meals is interesting. When I do professional speaking in front of large audiences, I will often ask 10 people in the audience to share what it is that they ate for supper last night. Invariably, 8 out of 10 will answer, "Oh, I had chicken" or "We had steak for dinner last night." And then I ask them what *else* they ate with their meat, and they say, "Oh yeah, rice/potato and a salad/veggie." When planning or eating a meal, we think of the meat as the primary food and the vegetables and starches as an afterthought.

In modern society, countries with meat-oriented cultures experience diseases that are almost non-existent in the rest of the world. The meat should be a condiment *(added in with the rest of the dish)* or a small part of the meal, maybe 3 to 4 ounces, while the starch and green vegetables should be the major part of the meal. Did you know that 3 to 4 ounces *(about the size of a deck of cards)* is actually what makes up one serving/portion of meat?

So, what is the answer? What is the ideal diet? Are you ready? *(I can hear you, you're saying, "Man, are we there yet? When will we get there? I'm hungry!")*

Let's talk about food, THE IDEAL DIET, also known as what your body was really made to eat before McDonald's or Burger

King arrived on the scene of the crime.

The World Health Organization recommends as the

IDEAL DIET:

70% 15% 15%

(Carbs) (Fat) (Protein)

NOT

The American Heart Association's

50% 30% 20%

(Carbs) (Fat) (Protein)

NOT

The Zone Diet's

40% 30% 30%

(Carbs) (Fat) (Protein)

NOT

what Atkins, Mayo, Grapefruit, Sugar Busters, etc., etc., etc.

ad nauseam says.

Daily Calories

People are usually confused about how many calories they should consume on a daily basis. They are usually equally confused about the amount they should eat and how to determine fat grams. Using the W.H.O. *(World Health Organization)* as our guide, here are the recommended calorie amounts for weight loss and weight maintenance.

A chart is the easiest teaching tool, so here it goes:

Calories for Weight Maintenance

Women	Men
1,600 daily	1,800-2,000 daily

Calories for Weight Loss

Women	Men
1,200 daily	1,300 daily

Now, using the chart to figure or calculate fat grams, we need to understand how many calories there are per one gram of: carbohydrate/protein/fat.

1 gram of carbohydrate has	4 calories
1 gram of protein has	4 calories
1 gram of fat has	9 calories
1 gram of alcohol has	7 calories

I call alcohol "Liquid Fat." There are 14 grams of alcohol in a jigger (shot), which is 1 1/2 ounces, happily giving you an instant 98 calories in that tiny little thing.

If the ideal <u>weight maintenance</u> diet should consist of 15% FAT daily, then we figure:

1,600 calories *(female)*		240 Fat Calories
x 15% Fat	**Then:**	÷ 9 calories / gram of Fat
240 Fat Calories		= 27 grams of Fat

So, if the ideal diet for <u>weight loss</u> for a female is 1,200 calories daily, then:

1,200 calories *(female)*		180 Fat Calories
x 15% Fat	**Then:**	÷ 9 calories / gram of Fat
= 180 Fat Calories		= 20 grams of Fat

This concept also can be used to figure gram amounts for carbohydrates and proteins. Now you know.

The Basics of My Recommended "Diet"

Note: I use the term "diet" in its original meaning, "the food that goes into your body on a daily basis," not in its more recently popularized meaning of "a short-term change in eating for weight loss purposes."

<u>**Women**</u> *(1,200 calories daily)*
Eat breakfast, lunch and dinner.
Have an afternoon snack and an evening snack.
Aim for no more than 20 grams of fat per day.
Drink 6-8 glasses of water each day.

<u>**Men**</u> *(1,300 calories daily)*
Eat breakfast, lunch and dinner.
Have an afternoon snack and an evening snack.
Aim for no more than 20 grams of fat per day.
Drink 6-8 glasses of water each day.

Weight Loss Plan Meal Options

On the following pages is the diet itself. It contains suggestions for healthy food items, sample menus, and portions for weight loss for women and men.

KEY:
T = tablespoon
t = teaspoon
c = cup
oz = ounce
I C B I N B = I Can't Believe It's Not Butter
WASA = name brand for a crunchy, cracker-like crisp bread high in fiber and fat free.

BREAKFAST OPTIONS *(9 to choose from)*:

1. The Cereal Treat:

4 oz soy milk, skim milk or 1% milk, almond milk
¾ c whole grain cereal *(Examples: Shredded Wheat Minis, any Kashi cereal, All-Bran, Raisin-Bran, Cheerios, or ¼ c Grape Nuts)*
Sliced fruits *(Mix small servings of three different kinds for variety, such as ¼ banana, ½ peach, 2 strawberries, ¼ c blueberries or 1 t. raisins)* or 1 fruit option

2. Cheese Toast:

2 slices 100% whole wheat bread, 1 ½ slices of WASA, or ½ whole wheat pita
1 oz cheese
1 fruit option

3. Egg McKaye:

(This breakfast should be eaten no more than twice a week.)

2 eggs or egg substitutes *(poached, hard boiled, soft boiled or scrambled, using Pam or olive oil)*
2 slices of 100% whole wheat bread, 1½ slices of WASA, or ½ whole wheat pita
1 fruit option

4. Bagel Break:

1 bagel *(preferably whole wheat or multi-grain)*
1 T. light cream cheese
1 fruit option

5. Peanut Butter Break:

1 ½ T. peanut butter *(Use "natural" peanut butter with the oil on the top, made without hydrogenated oils)*
2 slices 100% whole wheat bread, 2 WASA, 2 rice cakes or 1 whole wheat pita bread
1 fruit option (2 T. jam/jelly)

6. Weekend Treat:

2 six-inch pancakes *(preferably from the multi-grain pancake mix that many stores now carry)* OR 2 multi-grain waffles *(such as Kashi multi-grain frozen waffles)*
2 T. light syrup

8 oz skim milk

1 fruit option *(try sliced banana or blueberries on top of the pancakes/waffles, heated in the microwave for a few seconds)*

7. Power Shake: *(use blender)*

6 oz soy milk, skim milk, or 1% milk

1 medium banana or other fruit *(either frozen or fresh)*

Handful of ice

¾ c whole-grain cereal flakes or 1 packet of Medibase

8. Kool Breakfast:

8 oz low-fat vanilla yogurt *(try Dannon or Stonyfield Farms)*

¾ c whole-grain cereal

1 fruit option *(preferably sliced on top of the yogurt)*

9. Jamwich:

2 slices whole wheat bread or whole-grain bagel

1 T. light cream cheese

1 T. 100% fruit jam

LUNCH OPTIONS *(10 to choose from)*:

1. Chef's Salad:

1 oz cheese

2 oz chicken or turkey *(white meat only – baked or from the deli)* or fish *(boiled, baked or steamed but not fried)*

1 slice 100% whole wheat bread, 1 ½ slices WASA crackers or ½ pita bread

Any combination of: lettuce, cucumber, tomato, onion, or alfalfa sprouts

3 T. low-calorie *(light)* or fat-free dressing *(at 45 calories per tablespoon)*

1 fruit option or additional vegetable

HOMEMADE DRESSINGS

to try as an alternative to light store bought dressings:

Yogurt Sauce *(1 1/2 T. serving size)*:

1 T. plain yogurt, chopped green onions, ¼ t. dill and black pepper to taste

"Give Me the Flavor" Dressing:

1 t. soy sauce, 1 t. oil, 1 t. cumin, 1/2 t. garlic, 1/2 t. Worcestershire sauce, lemon juice and vinegar to taste

2. Sandwich:

3 T. bean dip or hummus and 1 oz cheese
– OR –
1 oz cheese & 2 oz lean meat *(such as chicken, turkey or fish)**
* *for chicken or turkey: use white meat only, baked or from the deli*
* *for fish: boiled, baked or steamed but not fried*
2 slices 100% whole wheat bread or ½ whole wheat pita
Lettuce and tomato
2 t. mustard *(brown or yellow)* or 1 t. light mayo or other condiment
1 fruit option

3. Dairy Meal:

8 oz low fat cottage cheese mixed with diced green onions, cucumbers, radishes, and tomatoes, topped with black pepper and dill
1 ½ slices WASA crackers *(crumble into mixture)*, 1 slice 100% whole wheat toast or 1 ½ rice cakes
1 fruit option

4. Kool Lunch:

8 oz low-fat vanilla yogurt
¾ c whole grain cereal *(e.g., Shredded Wheat Minis, any Kashi cereal, All-Bran, Raisin Bran, Cheerios, or ¼ c Grape Nuts)*
1 fruit option
Layer and stir to combine.

5. The Warm Up:

1 bowl or 2 c stew or hearty soup *(e.g., Bush Chili,
    Progresso Minestrone, Lentil, or Split Pea...look for low*
sodium options)
1 slice 100% whole wheat toast or 1 ½ WASA crackers
1 fruit option or vegetable

6. Potato Pleasure:

1 medium baked potato
½ c cottage cheese, beans, peas, soup or chili
– OR – 1 oz low-fat cheddar cheese
1 T. sauce *(A-1, salsa, Pickapeppa, etc.)*
1 fruit option or vegetables *(try chopped steamed broccoli on top!)*

7. Burrito Blow Out:

3 T. fat-free refried beans – OR – 2 oz chicken
1 large tortilla *(look for Mission whole wheat tortilla or
other brand)*
1 oz low-fat cheddar cheese *(shredded)*
Lettuce, tomato, salsa
1 apple

8. Hum *(no, not ham)* Burger:

3 T. hummus *(if you've never tried it, just give it a shot!)*
1 pita bread or 2 slices of 100% whole wheat bread
Sprouts, lettuce, tomato, brown mustard
1 fruit option

9. Tofu Sandwich: *(Try it once! Or better yet, get someone who likes it to show you how to make it!)*

4 oz grilled or sautéed tofu *(recommend using garlic, pepper, and light soy sauce)*
2 slices 100% whole wheat bread
Sauce of choice *(mustard, light soy sauce, ketchup, etc.)*
Lettuce, tomato
1 fruit option

10. Veggie Burger:

1 veggie burger *(try Garden Burger or Boca Burger or MorningStar)*
2 slices 100% whole wheat bread or whole wheat bun
Lettuce, tomato, pickles, as desired
Sauce *(optional)*
1 fruit option or vegetable
(Suggestion: sauté in pan with a small amount of olive oil rather that cooking in microwave)

AFTERNOON and/or EVENING SNACK
(Choose from below)

1. ½ oz cheese on whole-grain crackers, WASA, or 1 large rice cake
2. 1 rice cake with 1 ½ t. peanut butter, ½ t. honey or 1 t. light jam

3. 2 c light popcorn or plain, non-buttered popcorn with butter buds, Molly McButter, or spray margarine *(such as: "I Can't Believe It's Not Butter")*

4. 1 WASA cracker with 2 oz cottage cheese *(and maybe slices of cucumber!)*

5. fruit option or 1 frozen fruit bar *(look for "100% juice" on the package)*

6. 10 mini rice cakes, 1¼ large pretzels or 10 small pretzels *(try Quakes by Quaker)*

7. 1 cereal bar or granola bar of 140 calories or less *(some recommended brands are Kashi, Nature Valley, Kelloggs, and Luna)* **Best recommended afternoon snack.**

8. 1 Tootsie Roll Pop or 2 York Peppermint Patties *(I like them frozen!)* or even 2 small wrapped Dove chocolate pieces *(also frozen)*

DINNER OPTIONS:

These are not recipes but methods of combining different types of foods to make a balanced meal. The possibilities are endless, but as far as "what constitutes a balanced meal," here are some basic options. Note: Items A, B, C, and D are all part of the same meal.

(Choose one option from each category under A, B, C and D and then combine these options together to make a meal. Mix and match different options for endless variety.)

1. THE MEAT, STARCH, VEGETABLE COMBINATION

A) 3 oz chicken, 3 oz turkey, 3 oz fish, 8 medium shrimp – or – ¾ cup crabmeat *(flavor with any of the following: fresh garlic, lemon, ½ t cumin, dill, black pepper, basil or low-calorie sauces)*

B) ¾ c *(or 1 c for men)* cooked brown rice, pasta, corn, beans, lentils or other grains such as couscous or bulgar – or – 1 small baked potato

C) Cooked vegetables or 1 heaping soup bowl-sized raw salad *made with mixed greens, spinach, or lettuce (the greener the lettuce, the better) choose something other than Iceberg, which has fewer nutrients and vitamins than darker varieties).* Flavor with 3 T. low-calorie dressing or sprinkle 1 T. Parmesan cheese, 1 t. olive oil, and lemon.

D) 1 dessert, snack OR drink *(one alcoholic drink = 4 oz wine, 1 light beer, or 1 ½ oz liquor)*

2. MEATLESS MEAL *(This should be eaten at least once per week!)*

A) ²/₃ cup *(or 1 cup for men)* beans, peas or lentils

B) ²/₃ cup *(or 1 cup for men)* of a grain: rice *(preferably brown)*, pasta *(preferably whole wheat)*, corn or potato

C) Any amount of vegetables and/or a bowl of salad

D) 1 dessert, snack OR drink *(one alcoholic drink = 4 oz wine, 1 light beer, or 1 ½ oz liquor)*

3. *HEALTHY* FROZEN MICROWAVABLE MEAL

A)Healthy Choice, Lean Cuisine, Amy's, Kashi, Smart One's, etc. *(Any 350 calories or less)*

B) Bowl of salad or greens

C) 1 dessert, snack OR drink *(one alcoholic drink = 4 oz wine, 1 light beer, or 1 ½ oz liquor)*

WHAT IS A FRUIT OPTION?

Apple		1
Apple Sauce (Unsweetened)		1/2 cup
Apricots, fresh 2		
Apricots, dried 1		
Banana		1/2 or one small
Berries:	Black berries	1/2 cup
	Blue berries	1/2 cup
	Raspberries	1/2 cup
	Strawberries	3/4 cup
Cherries		10 large
Cider		1/2 cup
Dates		2
Figs, fresh		2
Figs, dried		3
Grapefruit		1/2
Cranberries (no sugar added)		1/2 cup
Grapes		12
Mango		1/2
Tangerine		1
Melon		1/4
Cantaloupe		1/4
Honeydew		1/4
Watermelon		1 cup
Nectarine		1
Orange		1
Papaya		1 cup
Peach		1
Pear		1
Persimmon		1
Pineapple		1/2 cup
Plums		2
Prunes		2
Raisins		2 tablespoons

50

SMALL TIPS THAT MAKE A BIG DIFFERENCE:

- Use water-packed tuna *(the rest have added fat from oil)*

- Take the skin off the chicken!

- Use light margarine, "I Can't Believe It's Not Butter," or Molly McButter instead of regular butter.

- Take a multi-vitamin daily.

- Sauces for meats or other foods add zip! Try new foods with your favorite sauces and you will probably like them. But caution: Use lightly. Some suggestions are: BBQ sauce, Worcestershire sauce, A-1 Steak Sauce, Pickapeppa, low-sodium soy sauce, Crystal Louisiana hot sauce, Indian curry paste, or any other sauce used lightly. Stay away from creamy sauces whenever possible,

- For issues with water retention *(only)*: Three times per day, for 3-4 consecutive days each month, mix 2 tablespoons of cold apple cider vinegar with ½ cups of cold water add Equal, Stevia or other artificial sweeteners.

THE INS AND OUTS OF PROTEIN

People talk about making sure they "get enough protein." Americans in general need not worry about eating enough protein. In fact, Americans in general eat too much protein...way too much protein. The amount of protein needed daily varies per person; it depends somewhat on body size and largely on the amount of activity you engage in each day. So if you are less active, you need to consume fewer grams of protein and fewer overall calories than someone who is more active.

Recommended Daily Amounts of Protein

<u>Children & Adolescents:</u>[1]

Children ages 1-3:	13 grams
Children ages 4-8:	19 grams
Children ages 9-13:	34 grams
Girls ages 14-18:	46 grams
Boys ages 14-18:	52 grams

<u>Adults:</u>

Women:	35-46 grams
Men:	35-55 grams
Pregnant Women:	60-70 grams
Pregnant Men: *(just seeing if you are paying attention here!)*	

Amounts of Protein in Foods:

½ c. cottage cheese	14 grams
8 oz yogurt *(Greek yogurt is 14-16 gms protein)*	10-11 grams
½ c. legume *(beans, peas, lentils)*	8 grams
8 oz milk *(no matter what fat content)*	8 grams
1 oz of meat, poultry, fish or cheese	7 grams
3 oz of meat *(about the size of a deck of cards)*	21 grams
1 egg	6 grams
½ c. oats	5 grams
1 T. peanut butter	4 grams
½ c. grain *(rice, corn, pasta, couscous)*	4 grams
1 slice bread	3 grams
½ c. potato *(white or sweet)*	3 grams
1 avg. sandwich slice of Swiss cheese	5 grams

Consider a 2 oz. turkey sandwich. Each slice of bread has

approximately 3 grams of protein. Two ounces of turkey, with seven grams of protein each, is 14 grams of protein *(2 oz. x 7 grams = 14 grams total)*. Add the 6 additional grams from the two slices of bread, and that makes a grand total of 20 grams of protein in one sandwich, about half of your daily protein needs *(not including that slice or two of cheese that you might have considered adding on)*. One slice of Swiss cheese adds another 5 grams of protein.

The average American *(male or female)* takes in 80 to 100 grams of protein daily...far beyond his or her real needs! Strange but true, folks. I believe these typical excessive amounts of protein are because America is such a meat-oriented society. Reducing the amount of protein and increasing the frequency of weight-bearing *(walking)* exercise should dramatically reduce the incidence of osteoporosis. Additionally, I recommend eating green leafy vegetables and beans for good sources of calcium that are also moderate in protein and very low in fat.

A pregnant woman, who needs only 60 to 70 grams daily, is more likely to give birth to a 9, 10, or 11-pound baby if she consumes 100 or more grams of protein daily. A baby this large could result in a difficult birth. However, eating the right amount of protein, especially during the third trimester of pregnancy, is extremely important because that is when your baby will have its greatest brain cell development. Ladies, the best idea is: In the beginning of your pregnancy, keep a food record for one week and count protein amounts. You will then know if you are eating too much or too little protein and have a better sense of what and how you should eat. Go back and use the food record once every few weeks to make sure you are continuing to stay on track.

Portions: "The Truth Will Set You Free"

I have given you suggested amounts to go by. This is amazingly important. If you really want to lose weight, you have got to ask yourself: "How did I get so big? What amounts have I really been eating?" The truth will set you free. Be honest with yourself. These suggested total daily calorie amounts are not to deprive you or starve you. Instead, they will enable you to realize that you just do not need to eat as much as you have been eating. Remember that those "usual" amounts are probably what caused you to gain the extra weight in the first place. Focusing on and becoming aware of your amounts is incredibly important. Because this is a high fiber, high starch, blood-sugar leveling diet, you will likely not be hungry between meals! And if you are, you can appease yourself with one of the healthy snacks that were previously mentioned.

It would be wise to weigh and measure your food for the first few weeks on the program *(not for forever, just the first few weeks)*. As you saw in the "Meal Options" section, for supper I recommend only 3 ounces of meat, which is about the size of a deck of cards. You could also by a small inexpensive food scale at most grocery stores, in order to help you get a better sense of ounces and grams. For starches, using a measuring cup is very helpful. Have ¾ of a cup of one of the following: rice, pasta, beans, peas, potatoes, or corn. Do not go back for seconds of starches or meats. Amounts are incredibly important with these food types. Note that I am not endorsing staying away from them all together.

When it comes to green and yellow vegetables *(broccoli, asparagus, green beans, English green peas, squash, zucchini, salads, etc.)*, you can really eat all you want, not a problem. Going back for seconds of these foods is fine.

If you decide to have a meatless or vegetarian meal one evening, it will look as if you have more on your plate because the starches spread out. Have $2/3$ of a cup of a legume (*any kind of bean, pea or lentil*) and $2/3$ of a cup of a grain (*rice, corn, or pasta*) and all the green or yellow veggies that you want. Still, the concept is to get used to lesser amounts.

"Healthy" frozen entrees are also a really good idea when you are first starting out on the program. Frozen meals give you instant portion control. You have heard of people paying big bucks to order frozen meals from various weight-loss companies. The best thing about these meals is that they are pre-portioned! Today, there is a plethora of excellent store-bought options available at most grocery stores: Healthy Choice, Lean Cuisine, Kashi, SmartOnes, and Amy's, to name a few. But remember that not all frozen entrees are good choices...other brands that are NOT geared toward the health-conscious can be packed with a surprising amount of fat and calories.

Those of you who have not discovered Amy's frozen food products are in for a treat. (*Of course, by touting their products, I am hoping the company will buy at least 100 of my new books, maybe more!*) But seriously, my family and I buy and eat them on a regular basis. My daughter's favorite easy meal to bring to campus with her is the Amy's individually-wrapped burrito (*which comes with or without cheese*). Amy's is one of the few companies that has actually brought some cultural diversity into its frozen cuisine. They offer Mexican, Italian, Indian (*my favorite!*) and American-style frozen entrees, mostly within 300 calories and 8 grams of fat. Take one with you for an easy lunch or eat it with a salad or steamed veggie for supper. It is frozen, so if you bring it to work in the morning and plan to eat it for lunch, you do not even need to store it in a fridge...it will be fine defrosting for a few hours.

Learning portions and amounts is necessary. Getting "use to" smaller amounts and learning to feel satisfied with less food is the key. You CAN learn new habits and behaviors!

Ask yourself: "What is really important to me? Do I want to eat what I want, when I want, all the time? Or do I want to become a normal-weight person?"

What do you really want?

I want alot of money!

SECOND STEP:

Boosting Your Metabolism Through Exercise and Diet Control

Many of us do not slow down with age, but unless we do something about it, our metabolisms will.

First, the bad news: At the ripe young age of 25, and sometimes earlier, your metabolism *(the rate at which you burn calories)* begins to slow down. In fact, it will decrease by about 8 percent every 10 years. So if you are 45, then your metabolic rate has slowed by 24 percent.

Now, the good news: There is no need to accept this fate! Your slowing metabolism is not a good excuse for throwing another hamburger on the grill or ravishing that frozen Snickers bar.

You CAN alter nature's course. Believe it! But don't rush around in search of the latest weight loss "wonder drug" or diet fad. Instead, pull your determination out of the closet and get down *(we are talking weight here)*. We need to change certain very specific habits in order to speed up our metabolic rate.

Eating Breakfast: The First Method for Speeding Up Your Metabolism

Do you skip breakfast? Be honest. Sometimes? All the time? Raise your newspaper if you skip breakfast. Ok, thanks, put it down. Now did you know this: If you consume 25 percent of your day's calories at breakfast, then you will "jump start" your metabolism.

I don't care if you are hungry or not, if you don't like breakfast, or if you don't like getting hungrier later in the day because of eating breakfast. You need to eat breakfast! You may need to start out small in order to get used to it *(especially if you tend to feel nauseous in the morning)*, and it may take one to two weeks of eating breakfast to realize, "Hey, I *do* feel like eating breakfast...in fact, I feel *better* because of eating breakfast!"

By doing so, you kick start your metabolism. The earlier you eat, the sooner your metabolic rate revs up. Yet, most people who are overweight don't eat breakfast. Right? Admit it. So, if lunch is your first meal of the day, that is when your metabolism finally begins to increase. It slows down the most at night, to conserve energy, but do you want it to keep "sleeping" until 12 p.m., even though you get up at 7 a.m.? No, you want it to get up when you get up and have it start working for you! I have some clients who do not eat breakfast *or* lunch, so their metabolism does not finally get going until the evening. Then they "graze" for dinner or eat one meal a day, from 6 p.m. to 10 p.m. Need I say more?

Consuming a glass of juice or a piece of toast is not enough. Your metabolic rate is slowest between 3 a.m. and 5 a.m., so the sooner you eat breakfast after waking up, the earlier your metabolism starts climbing. Increasing your metabolic rate will help to burn more calories. So, **EATING BREAKFAST CAN HELP YOU TO LOSE WEIGHT!**

Eating Routinely: (Three Meals Daily, Consistent Amounts, Regular Time)
The Second Method for Speeding Up Your Metabolism

I know we already discussed the need for routine meals, but it is crucial to understand that when you eat and how much you eat also affect your metabolism. ROUTINE MEALS don't just help you to control your appetite, hunger, and emotions, they ALSO HELP YOU TO SPEED UP YOUR METABOLISM. I cannot emphasize enough how important this is for successful early and long-term weight loss. When you have three, five, or even seven meals daily with the right *(same)* amount, at around the same time *(such as breakfast at 7 a.m. or 8 a.m., lunch at noon or 1 p.m., an afternoon snack at 4 p.m. or 5 p.m., and supper at 6:30 p.m. or 7:30 p.m.)*, then your body begins to trust when you will feed it and give off calories as opposed to storing them. Your body becomes a fine-tuned machine with the fuel coming in and going out on a regular schedule, allowing the machine to run at its highest level of efficiency. Yes! Sign up here! This is more important than most of us realize, so give it a try. Do it for one lousy month. Make the major effort to create a routine, stick with it, and see what happens.

Your body will become very efficient at burning calories if it is provided with nourishment on a consistent schedule. However, if you eat lunch much later than normal, have a larger lunch because you are starving, or eat a large afternoon snack, you throw your body off schedule. Then, your body does not know when the next meal is coming, so it holds onto *(stores instead of burns)* whatever calories you consume. And who wants to be a storehouse for calories? No one I know!

Many people who battle their weight tend to have very little routine in their eating schedule. This should be the first change that you make toward adopting a healthier lifestyle.

Walking: **The Third Method for Speeding Up Your Metabolism**

If you briskly walk *(3-4 miles per hour)* a minimum of five times a week for eight weeks in a row, you will speed up your metabolism. Hear me out. One hundred years ago, when your family was living in Boston, your great granddad walked eight blocks to his job *(in the snow, up hill both ways)*, worked all day in the same factory, then walked back home. It was called "transportation." Two hundred years ago, people would walk from their homes in outlying towns into Boston to go to a dance. Today, most forms of walking we call "exercise."

Today, we try to park our vehicles as close to the front door of our office as possible. Nurses, school teachers, even people who work outdoors, tell me that moving around at work in hallways is considered exercise. Yet, they still are 50-100 pounds overweight. Their bodies are used to this type of movement, so it is not challenging enough. They need to do more.

Speed walking or slow jogging are among the best exercises for burning fat and are simple too. You can do them with or without equipment and with or without a gym membership. Get out of the house, and just do it. It is hard to get yourself out the door, but once you are done, you will feel better about yourself and also more energized.

Exercise physiologists have demonstrated that you can speed up your metabolism by brisk walking 3 to 4 miles per hour (mph), preferably closer to 4 mph. You can begin slowly, at a pace that works for you, and gradually work up to your goal. The key is to gradually challenge yourself more and more.

For more details, see the next chapter.

Walking: Your Golden Ticket

Walking is the most important form of exercise for weight loss. With the right methods and the right routine, walking will get you where you need to go *(in more ways than one)*.

Aspects to consider: 1) When, 2) Where, 3) Speed, 4) Frequency, 5) Method of walking, 6) Stretching, 7) Shoes & shoe inserts, 8) Clothing and, 9) Water *(fluid replacement)*.

When to Walk

Ask yourself: "When is the best time for me to do this?" Look at your day and your responsibilities. Do you have children? What age? Can they be left alone? Do you have to pick them up at daycare or an after-school program, or can your mother-in-law do it? Are you married? Can your spouse watch the kids while you go for a walk? Where do you live? Is it safe, well-lit? If not, where else could you go? Are you a morning person? Can you get up early before everyone else and walk, or should you walk after work before you go home? Is your only time to walk late in the evening? Are you too tired then? Are you better off walking before or after a meal?

Personally, I think it is best to walk in the morning, before work or school. Then it is done, out of the way. You won't have to think about it later. Also, because your 30 minutes of exercise decreases stress for the next 1 ½ hours, you will be better able to handle whatever "hits the fan" at work. I also recommend, unless you have problems with low blood sugar, walking before breakfast. You'll walk harder.

Normally, it is difficult to walk during the day, say at lunchtime, yet that is OK, too. Many of my clients get two 15 minute breaks during the day, so they want to walk twice, for two 15 minute periods. The problem with this is that it does not speed up your metabolism enough, and you do not burn fat when you break that 30 minute walk in half.

Here is the deal: During the first 10 minutes of a 30 minute walk, you are burning carbohydrates in the liver for energy. I call this "stoking the fire." Then, for the next 20 minutes, you are burning fat. To boost the metabolism, you need that full 30 minutes.

Here is another option: If you can not walk in the morning before work, take your walking clothes and shoes with you. Right after work, change your clothes, go outside your office building, turn left or right, and walk *(make it automatic, don't give yourself time to think about whether or not you should do it)*. Or, change your clothes at work and then drive to a nice, safe, preferably flat area *(a high school track for example)*, or a gym *(if you can afford it/prefer being inside)*, and walk. Or, change your clothes at work and drive home, but don't go inside before walking. If you go inside, the rest is history, and you probably will not wind up walking. If you have to walk in the evening, I think it is better to walk before supper. Again, then it's done. If you walk after supper, it may be difficult to make it an exercise walk because you are full or sleepy.

Where to Walk

Where to walk? Definitely not in your former spouse, girlfriend or boyfriend's neighborhood! If you really have a lot of weight to lose, you want the least challenging situation, so go wherever the land is flat and the cars, dogs, and bill collectors are few.

Think pleasant neighborhoods; safe downtown sidewalks; high-school tracks; safe, shady, wooded areas; parks or community centers; and indoor tracks. One of my female clients likes the college track nearby. I said, "Makes sense to me...it's safe, well-lit, convenient..." And then she added, "Yeah, and what motivates me are the men's shorts." Some of my clients who travel always stay at hotels with gyms. Some bring their I-pods and walk the hallways in the hotel. Whether or not you have a gym membership, you CAN find a place to go walking. Just put your thinking cap on and do a little research into your local resources.

Treadmills, Gyms and Sports Clubs

Owning your own treadmill is a great idea. Then, there is no excuse not to exercise *(unless you cannot find your treadmill under all of the clothes you have hung on it)*. Seriously, I like the idea of the treadmill. With a home treadmill, weather, darkness, being alone *(safety)*, etc. won't be a problem *(unless of course, you didn't pay the utility bill on time)*. A basic treadmill, without all the bells and whistles, is fine. If you are taller or heavier *(above 250 lbs)*, then a longer, wider belt, and maybe a 2.5 HP treadmill is the way to go. Costs usually range between $400 and $700 *(probably comes out to less than one year's gym membership)*. HOWEVER, a) you can check out used sports stores *(like Play-It-Again Sports)*, garage sales, or the newspaper to see if you can find a used one, and b) if you purchase one and realize, for some foolish reason, that your treadmill is becoming an armoire, the treadmill has the best resale value of most any piece of exercise equipment. *(But hey, don't sell it, use it, for Pete's sake!... and who is Pete anyway?)*

Speed of Walking

Yes, the brisker the better, but begin slow *(2.5 mph)* and gradually increase your speed over time. Eventually, if you can increase your speed to 3.5 to 4 mph, that would be great. Depending on your current fitness level, you may need to begin with walking for only few minutes, maybe five, then eight the next day, then 10 to 12 minutes. Build up to 30 minutes, which is the minimum amount of time needed to speed up your metabolism. If you can gradually keep increasing it to 40 to 45 minutes, that would be really great. Over the years, some of my clients who really got into the walking increased their time to an hour. But their speed usually diminished over that period of time, and they lost the benefit. So I suggest that you "max out" at 45 minutes.

Frequency of Walking

Some people say walking is like sex, you can't do it enough. Exercise physiologists have found that walking a minimum of five out of seven days per week for eight weeks is enough to speed up the metabolism. But walking six or even seven days a week is, of course, even better. Sometimes people play a little game with themselves, or with a partner *(another great idea)*, to see how many days in a row they can walk. Eight? Nine? It will help to challenge you.

Burning Fat

Remember: During the first 10 minutes of walking, you are burning CARBS *(glycogen, fuel)* from the liver that your body then converts to get ready for fat burning. So, by walking 30 minutes, you will have 20 minutes of fat burning. If you walk for 40 minutes, you will have 30 minutes of fat burning.

Method of Walking

At first, you may feel weird doing it, but the best method or technique for walking for exercise is to SWING YOUR ARMS ACROSS YOUR BODY, not along your sides. This is the same motion you would use if jogging. When you jog, your arms naturally swing across the body. Try it where you are, right now. Your right arm reaches forward toward your left *(leading)* foot. This gives you balance. Then with the next step, your left arm moves forward toward your right foot, which is now in front. Watch a jogger or even jog for 10 feet *(if you can)* and you will notice how your arms naturally move.

This "arms across the body" technique will allow you to tighten your stomach, tighten your chest muscles *("pecs" or pectoralis major)*, and thin the underside of your arms *(triceps – the muscles many women show concern over when discussing "flabby arms")*. Yes, this technique works all three of these areas. *(See, and you thought you knew how to walk!)* It may feel a little awkward at first, or you may even feel slightly embarrassed, but this is the method needed to speed walk your way to losing weight and toning your body. Any initial embarrassment will wear off real quick as soon as the pounds start dropping.

Stretching

Yes, yes and yes. Some might say, "I'm not flexible enough to stretch." This is an oxymoron, is it not? We all need to stretch. Our muscles need to be stretched. The truth doesn't need to be stretched, just the leg muscles, to help you walk in comfort. Stand on the tips of your toes on a stair *(holding onto a handrail)*. Let your heels sink below your toes, and you will stretch your calves, which will also help prevent shin splints. A great book to check out is *Stretching* by Bob and Jean Anderson.

Apparel : More Important Than You Think
Shoes and Shoe Inserts

Use common sense and go to an independently owned shoe store where the sales person knows how to fit the right shoe to your foot. Getting a shoe that fits right is really important. Probably the most important piece of clothing you can own is a comfortable, well-fitted pair of walking shoes. Often, it may be even better for your foot to buy a shoe that is a little bigger than what you would normally buy. One caveat is, when you really begin losing weight, you may need smaller shoes and clothes. Yes! You may also want to try shoe inserts such as those by Orthotics or Dr. Schols.

Clothing

Layered clothing is a good idea. As you warm up, you can remove the outer layers. Be sure your clothes are flexible as well. Exercising in jeans is not a good idea. Wear clothes you are comfortable in and have the most range of motion in. Buy good socks.

Drinking Water

Drink before you walk, use the bathroom *(do I sound like your mother again?)*, then drink more water. If you live in a hot climate, take a bottle of water with you *(or two bottles, which can then double as added arm weights)*. Soon you will "become the bottle."

Do You Have Trouble Walking?
Try Water Walking!

If you cannot walk on land because your feet are bad or your knees are killing you, it is time for "Plan B"...water walking! I am not talking about water aerobics. Water aerobics is terrific exercise, but it mostly tones and strengthens your muscles and does less for helping you lose body fat.

If you get into a pool of chest-high water and regularly walk for 20 minutes in the shallow end *(or in a lap pool, which has no deep end)*, you can lose weight until you are able walk on land. How is this? There is a 12 times greater resistance against the body in water than on land. You will be moving slower, but working harder as you do it *(with less pressure on the joints)*. One 435-pound client *(who lost 235 pounds in three years!)* "water walked" for her first year on my program. She lost 115 pounds by going to the pool five days a week and walking. It taught me that where there is a will, there is a way!

There were additional positive outcomes to her life that I will mention later. Where to water walk? If you do not have a pool, check out a gym with a pool if you can afford one, or for a less expensive/free option, find a YMCA or community recreational center near your home or place of work.

Why Walking Burns Fat the Best

I knew you were going to ask. I mean here you are, one who loves the Stairmaster, lifting weights, swimming, or the reclining bicycle, and are thinking, "What does walking do for weight loss that these other exercises don't?"

Well, here it goes. When you do aerobics, bicycle, or high-level Stairmaster, your breathing rate increases to about 65% of what your normal breathing rate is. Your body then needs quick energy, so it goes to the liver to burn glycogen, which is stored carbohydrates. But you want to burn fat, right? When you walk briskly, your breathing rate is only 50% greater than that of your normal breathing rate, unlike the other previously mentioned exercises. Therefore, your body will burn CARBS for about the first 10 minutes but then switch to burning FAT. So, walking is among the best fat-burning exercises.

When you swim *(unlike water walking with a higher resistance)*, the water temperature is usually colder than the body temperature. In order to prevent hypothermia *(body temperature lowering below normal)*, the body holds on to body fat and burns carbohydrates *(glycogen)* as its primary source of energy. So for this reason, swimming is not a good fat-burning exercise.

A Word on Weights: WAIT!!!

Do not lift weights *(barbells, dumbbells, etc.)* in the beginning of your weight loss journey. When you are starting a weight loss program, especially "youse guys" *(the men)*, your testosterone says to you, "I must build muscle or Mr. Schwarzenegger will call me a girlie mon." Hold your testosterone at bay for just a moment, gentlemen.

By walking, using portion control, and making good food choices, you will lose weight. As you begin to do so, you will get psyched and motivated to commit to making this new routine into a lifestyle, and you can *then* begin your mission to become Mr. Atlas, The Hulk, or whichever big-muscled hero you admire. This goes for you ladies as well.

The problem with weight training is that the muscle you build is denser and therefore heavier, than fat. With weight training, you get on the scale, and you find that you are a few pounds heavier one week *(from gaining muscle mass)*. You may then become discouraged, decide that "it's never going to happen anyway," and think everything this Dr. Freddy Kaye guy says is a bunch of bologna...and we don't want that.

You might say, "But anyone in their right mind recognizes that if their clothes are looser, they must be losing weight, even though the scales say they are heavier, right?" Unfortunately, this is often not the case. Most of us focus primarily on the almighty scale as the end-all, be-all, especially when we are first trying to lose weight. *(This is not good!)* Using the scale as your *only* measure of accomplishment in your weight loss journey can be detrimental to your self-motivation. *Don't forget about how you are feeling, how your clothes are fitting, and your slowly increasing fitness level!*

Psychologically, you may be momentarily devastated because you thought that you were doing well, but the scale doesn't concur. So, my suggestion is to stay away from the weights for a little while, maybe two to four months. Get a head start on weight loss through speed walking and eating right, increase your motivation, and then start thinking about using light weights at frequent repetitions. But whatever you do, don't quit walking.

Ladies: Many of you may be concerned with some extra flab *(pardon me)* under the arms. Listen carefully. By swinging the arms while walking you will diminish the underarm fat in the triceps area. Later, by lifting some light weights in exercises that target the triceps muscles *(get any trainer to show you how to do the exercise with the proper technique)*, you will make good progress on the arms and turn flab into muscle!

So wait on weights, in general, because they can become psychologically and physiologically self-defeating in the short term.

A Reminder on Exercise for Older Individuals

In the early 1990's, Tufts University's Institute on Aging conducted an exercise study with people in their 70s, 80s and 90s. The study, at their facility in Boston, took 100 people and measured their stamina and strength as baseline. They then put all of these participants on a program for three months, designed to enhance their strength and stamina. The program included a walking program, treadmills, machines and weight training. At the end of the three months *(not very long!)*, they re-measured the participants and found that each of them had experienced a minimum increase of 50 percent in strength and stamina, even the 90 year olds!

The evidence is clear. Your body wants to be taken care of. It needs routine or continual movement to strengthen itself and to prevent degenerative diseases that can be minimized or even avoided. Of course, the longer you let your body go into "disrepair," the more difficult it will be to get it back into shape. But it is not impossible! If you have a plan or a program in which you gradually increase your frequency of aerobic activity *(i.e. walking, jogging, strength training)*, you will improve in these areas. And remember, 30 minutes of exercises decreases stress for 1½ hours. I say it's worth it!

THIRD STEP:

Changing Your Habits and Behaviors

So you want to lose 30 pounds by Friday at noon? Sounds nice, I know, but let's get realistic. We all have our individualized eating habits that we have developed for all kinds of reasons. Some of those habits are good, but many are not so good. We could blame anyone. Some excuses I have heard are: "My parents made me clean my plate" or "If I ate my vegetables, I got ice cream for dessert. Now that I can eat ice cream whenever I want..."

Or even worse: "My spouse is always late for dinner, so I snack while standing in the kitchen...Maybe if I stand up, I'll get fat toes instead of a wide waist..." Yeah, right.

When you arrive home, which room do you gravitate to first? The kitchen of course! You go straight to the refrigerator door "just to check it out" and make sure everything is still there, especially because you have a teenage son who invades the kitchen frequently.

You need to step back and honestly look at your true eating habits. Sit down with a journal or notepad and write five reasons why you are overweight. Seriously...go get a pen and paper...I'll wait. Some examples are:

1. Boredom
2. Frustration
3. Anger
4. Laziness or lack of energy
5. Emotional eating
6. Reward

Becoming aware of why you have become overweight leads to the next step: changing your habits and behaviors.

Enough Is Enough!

Say this to yourself: "Enough is enough! I want to take better care of me. I deserve a better me. I take care of everyone/thing else in my life *(job/family/ bills/parents/kids...)*. Now, I need to take care of me!"

As a friend of mine says, "It's about damn time!"

You must always keep in mind the concept of BALANCE.

Slow Down Your Eating

It is likely that your mother told you, at some point *(or every single night at the dinner table)*, to put your fork down between bites of food. But I ask 'ya...whoever really listened to their mother's good advice? Well, she was right, in a sense. Many people load food into their mouth, begin chewing, and then immediately reload the fork and shove in another bite while still chewing the previous bite. Sounds vulgar almost when you stop and think about it, but look around, and you will see what a common practice this is. In this manner, your fork is constantly "cocked and ready to go." This habit will not help you learn to eat slower or eat less food. Many of us do not even realize that we do this. However, there is an easy solution.

Rule #1: Make a commitment to yourself, "While I am chewing, I will not put more food on my fork. I must wait until I am completely finished chewing before 'reloading'."

You don't have to set your fork down and place your hands in your lap *(unless, of course, your mother is watching)*, just don't reload it. However, after living in the South for many years, I have been told that setting your fork down between bites is, in fact, considered proper manners. So you may want to improve both your manners and your eating habits in one swift step!

Rule #2: In the middle of the meal, stop eating for one minute.

This will give your stomach time to say "hello" to your brain and inform it that it is beginning to get full. The only downside to this excellent technique is that your spouse or partner *(more often than not, a husband)* takes it as a sign that you have finished and quickly negotiates his fork to your plate. A light slap on the hand is appropriate.

Once you have committed the first two rules to memory and have begun successfully applying them, you may venture out to Mental Rule #3, an eye-opening experience and the ultimate test of dexterity!

Rule #3: For one week at dinner, eat with your fork in your opposite hand!

If you are a "righty" eat "lefty." If you are a "lefty" eat "righty." And if you happen to be even less dexterous than you had imagined, there is always the option of using a bib! *(As long as it is one that does not catch food and provide you with leftovers!)* But by all means, do not try the bib idea in a restaurant *(unless, of course, you are having lobster!)* and please do not send me your dry cleaning bill. The increased dexterity will come in handy one day, when you least expect it!

To review, slow down your eating with the Three Rules:

1. Wait until you are finished chewing to put more food on your fork.
2. In approximately the middle of a meal, stop eating for one minute.
3. For one week at dinner, eat with your fork in the opposite hand that you normally use.

These behaviors will force you to become more aware, to slow down your eating, to give your body more time to recognize when it is full *(before it is "too late")* and to eat less food.

Sit Down to Eat

Situation #1: "The Pre-Dinner Dinner"

Many people often stand up in the kitchen to snack, particularly prior to supper or late in the evening. Maybe you just arrived home from work…you feel hungry and do not know what you are going to do for dinner. You gravitate to the snack food and begin munching while you think about it. Even if no one else is there to see you, standing in the kitchen and munching still counts as calories!

Situation #2: "The Never-Ending Taste Test"

You are cooking a dish, say a beef stew *(that you have made 5,200 times before, to be exact!)*, and you need to taste it as you add ingredients. While determining what to add more of, you decide that neither the tasting finger nor a teaspoon is big enough to give you the full effect. So you use a large spoon and begin losing track after the 15th "taste test." By the time you sit down to eat your meal, you realize that you are, strangely, not as hungry anymore, but you fix yourself a normal-size portion anyway. By the time you finish it, will you have consumed a total of one and a half portions? Two? Probably more than you initially meant to.

Situation #3: "The Office Party"

You find yourself at an evening office party with a wonderful spread of food. You cruise the table, with the intention of taking a few tastes "here and there." However, you soon realize that you have basically eaten a full meal while standing. You don't remember what you ate or even making the conscious decision to do so. Even worse, five different people have said "hello" to you at the table, shook your hand *(who knows where their hands have been?)*, and you have continued sticking your hand into that yummy finger food. Yikes! And maybe it is even worse and you have got broccoli sticking out of your teeth!

This is alternative to standing at the hors d'oeuvre table and eating until you have lost track of what you ate: Peruse the table, stake out your options, and try take a mental note of which foods may be the lower-fat and therefore wiser choices. Then, grab a plate, take a reasonable amount of food, and find a place to sit down. This way, you will have a chance to be aware of what and how much you are eating, and you will probably even enjoy it more as well. This is also an excellent method for use at a family reunion or a social gathering such as at a pot luck meal. Carefully consider the spread, get a plate, make wiser, low-fat choices, take small portions, and then sit down and eat. You will eat less this way.

Once I was at a large birthday party with tables upon tables of gourmet food. The place was packed, so there were few chairs and almost no eating tables set up for guests. Upon getting my plate together, I looked around at the crowded situation. Right then, I noticed a stairwell leading upstairs, so I sat on one of the steps *(yes, in my fine blue suit)* and dined on the staircase. "How crass," you might think...but within minutes, the staircase was filled with elegantly dressed women and men, dining on their gourmet goodies. I had started a trend, and it caught on beautifully. *(Of course, had it not, I would have enjoyed my food just as much.)*

The Daily Diet Record

Eighty-five percent my clients who keep a daily journal of what they eat lose weight. Fact or fiction? FACT!

Probably the most important tool in successful weight loss is **WRITING DOWN WHAT YOU PLAN ON EATING BEFORE YOU EAT.**

The keyword is BEFORE. This is quite important in learning to "think before you act," to analyze a food situation before you get stuck in it. Some major weight loss companies recommend using a food journal *after* you have finished eating, but I believe that in order to change one's eating habits, you must become aware of what you do before you do it, to *think before you act.*

I have included a sample page of the Daily Diet Record in the chapter titled "Daily Diet Record and Sample Menu" that you can copy and then use to begin recording what and when you eat. Try to be honest with yourself. This is for no one but you. Write down everything you eat. By learning to analyze the food environment ahead of time, you can make lower fat choices and use better portion control. Otherwise, "the rest is history."

For example: It is lunchtime and you are "starving," so you automatically pull into the familiar fast food drive-through. Immediately upon arriving, the friendly, crackly little voice in the box inquires, "Welcome to _____. What would you like to order?" You had not yet arrived at that momentous decision, so as you nervously fumble for a complete thought, the old habits kick in and you blurt out, "I'd like a cheeseburger, fries and a soda." The voice box replies, "Is that a large soda and large fries?" "Sure," you sheepishly reply. And before you know it, the little voice in the box is suddenly a person handing you a greasy, fattening, high caloric, high sugar meal that is someone wanting to lose weight's *(or be healthy)* worst nightmare.

No planning, no thought – just the usual reaction. Then of course later in the day, since you know you have "blown it" already, you think, "Why not have a candy bar from the snack machine? What's the difference?"

Thankfully, this is not real life *(at least not today)*, so we can rewind this tape. Let's start from the beginning: Before getting into your vehicle to drive off for lunch, you think about where to go and what to get. Maybe you realize that Wendy's is next to McDonald's and that there, you could get a baked potato with taco sauce and a salad for lunch. So, when you get into your car, before even leaving, you write that down in your daily food diary *(could be a copy of mine or one you make up yourself)*. When you arrive at your point of destination, you know what you are going to order and you have already planned it out. You feel good about yourself for making a good food choice. Later, for an afternoon snack, you grab one of those cereal snack bars that you brought from home. Control. You are now in control, a good feeling. You thought before you acted.

Planning meals is a very important habit. You must analyze where you will be and what food will be available. What time will you eat? How do you need to plan for it? Should you bring lunch or a snack to work with you? Will you be in a meeting where the meal is ordered out? If so, will you have a say in what is ordered?

Control. You want to control your eating environment. You do not want it to control you.

Self Analyze and Be Honest

At the end of each week, take an honest look at your Daily Diet Record *(by the way, for an easy and cheap way to do it, you can just buy a small 3" x 5" memo pad to use as your Daily Diet Record)*.

Self analyze, ask yourself these questions:
- What did you eat?
- Where were you?
- What time did you eat?
- What was the situation?
- Were you alone, with friends, on a date?
- Were you bored, sad or angry?
- How were you feeling at the time?
- Were you "food congratulating" yourself?
- Did you make good choices?
- Did you wait so late to eat that you overate or made the wrong choices?

Check it out! You may think, "I know what I eat everyday! I don't need to write that down!" But it is hard to gain insight into your behaviors when you make so many choices every day, sometimes without even taking the time to think about them. This exercise will allow you to take a step back and become aware of and analyze your food-related behaviors in a way that you have never before done.

See what your patterns are, for better or for worse. See when you make good choices and when you make bad choices. Notice what the situations were at those times. Then, objectively try to think of other choices that you could have made or how you can change the situation next time, without being down on yourself. This is not about keeping score, this is about analyzing yourself and learning what factors influence the decisions that you make. Keep learning from this record, and you will continuously get better at losing weight.

This is a process, a direction on the path, a learning situation. It is NOT an all or nothing, be perfect or fail diet!

Pre-Plan, Pre-Shop and Pre-Cook

When you are ready to eat, you will be able to be in control and make wise choices only if you have the correct food available to you. If not, you will grab "whatever is there." Being hungry, making poor choices, then feeling out of control and guilty, is not good! Let's work together to change that.

The concept of "batch cooking" or pre-cooking in bulk is an excellent technique. Do this most every week, a few times per week. Once you begin to batch cook on a regular basis, "whatever is there" will no longer be beef-a-roni/ramen noodles/leftover pizza but will instead become healthy food staples that can be easily morphed into a variety of different dishes.

An example from my personal life: On Sunday evening, I batch cook whole-grain pasta, brown rice, new or baked potatoes, and frozen beans, such as lima beans. I add a little seasoning *(dried herbs, garlic, pepper, or a salt substitute - stay away from lots of salt)* and stick them in the fridge. I then have separate "batches" of starches in large plastic containers in the fridge, ready to go when I am ready to eat. You can do the same with chicken breasts *(skinless, boneless)* or alternatively, get your local grocery store deli to cook you chicken or turkey breasts. You pick up the food on your way home from work and "voila!" *(there it is)* in your fridge.

There are many different ways to combine these food staples, and you may need to get creative or get ideas from other people to figure out how. For instance, with a pot of brown rice pre-cooked, one night you could make a simple chicken and rice dinner *(and add a green vegetable and a salad)*, and the next night, you could go Southern with black-eyed peas and rice or Latin with black beans and rice *(and of course a green veggie and/or salad)*. You can increase flavor by doing simple things such as sautéing garlic, onions and green pepper, then mixing the sautéed vegetables in with the black beans, and by topping your black beans and rice with some low-fat cheddar cheese and salsa. If you do not have time to soak and cook beans from scratch, using canned or frozen beans is an extremely quick way to go. When using canned beans, be sure to strain and rinse them to get rid of as much of the salt as possible, or buy low-sodium or no-sodium varieties if you can find them.

Now, with healthy basic foods available in your fridge or freezer there is no need to go for the cookies in the pantry come supper time. Take the food out of the fridge, put the right amounts on your plate *(the 8-inch Freddy Plate, which you will hear more about later)*, add sauces *(such as A-1, low-sodium soy, Worcestershire, balsamic vinegar, mustard or salsa)*, then place the excess food back in the fridge or freezer. Heat up your plate in the microwave *("nuke it," as my son says)*, add a green vegetable *(it can be fresh, frozen, or canned – just try to stay away from frozen or canned vegetables that have any added salt or butter – some do, many don't)*, sit down and slowly enjoy your supper.

You have now finished eating and the first word that pops into your mind is "seconds!" You want seconds? Eat as many green veggies or as much salad *(with low-calorie dressing)* as you want, but please, no seconds for the starch or meat. Remember, the slower you eat, the more likely you are to start feeling that "satisfied feeling" before you finish your plate and start pining after seconds. Remember:

EATING SLOWLY WILL HELP YOU TO FEEL MORE SATISFIED WITH LESS FOOD.

If you routinely batch cook, then you will have the right food available almost immediately. You will be in control and will be able to eliminate the pre-supper snacking, over-tasting while cooking, and grazing. Control! Yes!

By the way, a little off topic, but I would like to share with you a suggestion related to leftovers that I actually learned from - would you believe – my former mother-in-law. *(Who, by the way, happens to be terrific. My old saying is that I should have married my former mother-in-law instead of my former wife!)* Anyway, if there are leftovers that are really leftover and too far gone to eat or put in the freezer, but that you don't want to stink up the garbage can with, you can place the leftovers in a plastic container *(choose one you can't see through)* with a well-fitted cover, store it in the inside door of the fridge for a few days with any other table scraps and when it is full, get rid of it. Besides decreasing the stench of your trash can, it also lessens the possibility that you will eat the extra leftover food out of guilt. A more environmentally-friendly option is to create a compost pile in the ground, especially if you live in a wooded area or have a garden you could add it to.

A Different Way to Set Your Table

One of the easiest, most beneficial things you can do to decrease the amount you eat at meals is to use "The Freddy Plate." "The Freddy Plate," termed so by Mark, my nuclear physicist friend, is an eight-inch in diameter salad plate – perfect as your new supper plate! In America, the usual supper plate is 10 to 10 1/2 inches across. In Europe, the plate is usually 9 inches across. This may be one reason why Europeans are smaller than Americans *(more to follow)*...

Another useful idea is this: *(Are you ready to laugh at me?)* Eat with chopsticks! Yes, I mean the two sticks they serve in Asian restaurants that you hold together and use as a utensil, instead of a fork. It may sound weird, but only to those of us who are not of Chinese, Japanese, or other Asian descent. This will likely slow down your eating. You may be laughing *(so am I)*, but I am serious. Just a thought! Be open-minded and just give it a try. It takes practice, but it is not as hard as it looks or as it seems the first time you try to use them. Before you give up or resort to stabbing at your food, try asking someone to show you how to use the chopsticks the next time you go out for Chinese or sushi.

Okay, I am going to confess and get a little personal here...I actually use them at home...yes, for real. Yes, every night. No, I am not part-Asian. I realize that I am "a little different," but I started using them years ago and simply got hooked. Not only do I eat more slowly and thus, enjoy my food more, I also found that I actually prefer the taste and feel of the wooden chopsticks in my mouth more than the metallic taste of a hard metal fork. Just try it! It can't hurt! It is possibly the most fun weight loss technique you have ever tried!

Move On: The Show is Over, Don't Wait for the Encore

After a meal, leave the table immediately. Go brush your teeth to create a new flavor in your mouth, so you will not be as tempted to eat more. Then, come back and clean the kitchen. *(Or bribe, beg or coax someone else to do it!)* After dinner, make a real attempt to stay out of the kitchen for the rest of the evening *(except to refill the water glass that you should keep with you at all times)*.

Living Alone and Eating

Many of us who are single or whose children are out of the house enjoy reading or watching TV while eating. This is normal and should not necessarily be discouraged. Yet, to prevent unnecessary eating, you should put all extra food away before you sit down to eat *(except for the veggies that can remain out, ready for when that craving for seconds occurs)*.

Now, imagine this scenario *(which most of us have experienced at some point)*: During the middle of your favorite weekly sitcom, you finish eating the food on your plate. However, the show is still on! Naturally, you feel that you need more food in front of you to complete your program. This is trouble!

Remember: Keep only the veggies out. All the other food should have already been put away. Or, at the next commercial break, toss the plates *(gently, of course)* into the kitchen sink, brush your teeth, and then go back to the tube to continue "vegging out." We all have our guilty pleasures in life *(such as stupid TV shows)*, but we can make an attempt to minimize our guilty pleasures by not constantly pairing them together. For instance, watching TV in the evening before you go to sleep is not a sin...BUT eating constantly throughout your hour of shows, getting a snack in between each one, or watching TV instead of doing some type of daily physical activity is at least borderline sinful, as far as your waist is concerned.

Alternatives to Eating

Years ago, Dr. Kelly Brownell, in his LEARN Program, laid out a list of alternatives to eating.[2] He recommended having a list of other activities to do for the moment you begin focusing on food. Sure, you could always clean out the garage...but here is a better activity list, from Dr. Brownell, that you can use immediately *(along with my two cents on each one)*:

Walk the Dog - The dog will love it, and soon the dog will learn that between meals, you walking into the kitchen is the sign for "let's go for a walk!"

Call A Friend - Have a buddy, someone you can call in a moment for help or for companionship. Talk, complain, plan, schmooze, cry, or laugh *(or better yet, if you have a cell phone, talk to them while taking a walk)*.

Shop For Plants - You know you could use some, indoor or outdoor, on tiny apartment balcony or in big backyard, along with some new pots. Do you have a local nursery that is creative and a delight to stroll through? *(Don't know? Look in a phone book!)* Plants can uplift spirits, contently listen without interrupting, bring life to a dull room, and even fill your house with cleaner air! Simply amazing!

Take a Shower or Bath - In an instant, you step out of restrictive clothing and into a warm, delightful world. Stand there until you feel totally relaxed *(as long as someone else doesn't need to shower next)*. Or take a bath, and make it a big deal. Incorporate candles, music, a book and or bubbles *(or if all of the above are too flowery for you, settle for just a book/magazine)*. Where else can you feel so pampered?

Listen to Music - When is the last time you listened to "A Whiter Shade of Pale" by Procol Harem or Julie Andrews singing "The Rain in Spain" from "My Fair Lady"? Or how about your favorite rap or R&B artist, if that's your style? Smooth jazz? Norah Jones? You get the drift! Whatever makes YOU feel good. Especially if you are alone, sing out loud and off key, who cares *(unless you actually have the ability to sing on key, in which case you might as well go ahead and make the rest of us look bad!)*

Take a Drive - Jump in the car, open the windows, crank up the music and head toward the best "drive" in town. Cruise. Enjoy!

Read a Book - A mystery, if you like something intriguing. A non-fiction, if you want to be mentally stimulated or learn something new. A romance, if you want to take a mental trip to your heartland. A sexy book, if...well, whatever.

Do whatever *(healthy)* activity you need to do to take your mind off of food.

Of course, this does not include unhealthy activities like drinking, smoking, etc. No use in trading one unhealthy habit for another. There are many things we can do to control stress-induced or boredom-induced eating. In the heat of the moment, it is important to have a list of things that you can do instead of eating. It is important to make the list meaningful and personalized to fit your wants, needs, and desires. Consider posting it on the front of the fridge.

Some other examples are: learn something new, take a walk, prepare a budget or organize your finances, plan your weekend, ride a bike, make somebody happy, meet up with friends, visit a sick person, clean, put together that photo album you have been waiting a year *(or five)* to do, go swimming, play with your kids or someone else meaningful to you, keep a journal, catch up with relatives, send someone a card, grab a ball or frisbee and get outside, collect things, embroider, fix something that is broken, or go to a sports event. Now you come up with your own list.

The Splurge Meal: Yes, You Do Get to Reward Yourself

Here is another way of thinking that will help you really succeed in the long run: Six days a week, I ask you to be good. Make good food choices, choose the right amounts, and eat at routine times. But ON THE SEVENTH DAY, CHOOSE ONE OF YOUR THREE MEALS AS A "BLOWOUT MEAL." Eat whatever you want, within reasonable amounts. Yes, that is what I said – once a week, enjoy a Splurge Meal! Have reasonable amounts, so you don't get sick, but have anything you have really been dying to eat, and enjoy it without the guilt. Then the next meal, get back on track.

Note: This is called a Splurge MEAL, not a Splurge DAY. The next meal, you get right back on track. This gives you a reward for being good as well as a break from your new reality. The other important feature of the Splurge Meal is that it allows you to prove to yourself that you are actually in control of yourself and your behaviors. After doing this, you should feel more confident that the next time you "accidentally" have a Splurge Meal, you will be able to get yourself right back on track.

The Splurge Meal is especially useful with special occasions, eating out, or as a release. Once per week, it is there, available as your "release valve." This meal also includes a dessert. Go out to dinner at your favorite restaurant, enjoy dining with friends, or even sequester yourself at home with a terrific movie and your "drug of choice" (*i.e. pizza, fried chicken, or whatever "does it for you"*). It is your Splurge Meal, and you have earned it!

Tip: A Splurge Meal is most fulfilling when you plan it out and can look forward to it. For instance, if you know you have a dinner party over the weekend, plan ahead that that will be your Splurge Meal and look forward to it. Or, pick a certain night *(maybe over the weekend)* to go to your favorite restaurant and make that your Splurge Meal. The Splurge Meal is less fulfilling when you "slip up" and have an unintended Splurge Meal that you didn't even mean to have. So prevent accidental Splurge Meals and instead, plan and look forward to your purposeful once-a-week Splurge Meal. This way, you can enjoy yourself and feel proud of yourself for your success and discipline over the rest of the week.

Caution: You may really "blow it" on your first official Splurge Meal *(in other words, eat something or so much that it makes you feel sick)*, but if you do, you will know it *(heh, heh)* and hopefully not repeat the volume or heavy fatty choices that you made. Again, be careful of amounts. You may find that the food you were lusting for wasn't actually that fulfilling after all. It becomes a good realization and allows you to recognize that all unhealthy food is not tasty just because it is unhealthy. There are certain foods that you really like and want to treat yourself to occasionally and other foods that you could give up without really missing them. In the future, to possibly help you with portion size, you may decide to split that gooey, fatty dessert with someone else instead of adding it onto the rich Splurge Meal you just had. Or, if you are dining alone, just ask the person at the next table *(hey, just kidding)*.

Of the three daily meals *(breakfast, lunch and dinner)*, the best splurge meal is usually dinner. If you have breakfast as your Splurge Meal, it is sometimes difficult to get back on track for the rest of the day. Still, it is your choice and up to you. Another option is just a particularly decadent Splurge Dessert, instead of the whole meal.

Ironically, a person's first experience with the Splurge Meal is often the worst; people usually overindulge and feel guilty, but learn from it. Then, we get better in what and how extravagantly we splurge. Some save the Splurge Meal as their "just in case" meal or their little "ace in the hole." But do NOT "save up" Splurge Meals for more than a week. In other words, don't tell yourself: "I haven't had a Splurge Meal in four weeks, so I'll just splurge on every meal for the next two days!" No. You don't want to go there. When it comes to a Splurge Meal, earn it and then enjoy the splurge. Then, with the next meal, immediately get yourself back on track. The first time you are able to do this successfully, you will feel good about yourself and have a new found appreciation for your own ability to control what you eat.

Forget the Guilt

The Splurge Meal is set up not only to reward you, but to help you realize that it is okay to eat something "you shouldn't" every once in a while. Of course, the key words there are "every once in a while." You do not have to become resigned to never again be able to eat your favorite unhealthy foods...you just need to make sure they are not a part of your regular diet. This program is set up so that if you lose your way, you can always get back on it. When you are on the program, you will do well. However, when you "blow it" *(I say "when" instead of "if" because all of us "blow it" sometimes)*, it is not "all over." It is not a big deal. It is not the end of the world *(or your chance at losing weight)*. Just recognize what you did wrong, decide specifically how you are going to try to prevent it from happening next time, and then get back on the program, The Physician's Nutritionist.

WEIGHT LOSS CAN NOT BE ALL OR NOTHING.

One way that this program is different from some of the others is that I will never say "Never." I will never say that you can never eat a certain food. I will certainly never say that you can never eat a certain food group. This program is about taking the direction toward a new lifestyle. And since changing our lifestyles is not an easy thing to do, you must recognize that you will slip up and that when you do, you can always just pick yourself up and get back on this Path.

Guilt is something we all have. Catholics think Catholic guilt is the worst, Baptists think theirs is the worst, and Jews think that theirs is the worst kind of guilt. But the truth is that it is all the same guilt: you must do this and this or else such and such will happen. The guilt does not have to be there. Guilt can very easily lead to low self-esteem and depression. It does not need to be there. Instead, replace it with a conscious, purposeful decision to do better. When you mess up, remember: Just get back on the program.

Whenever people "go on a diet" they expect themselves to be perfect. How many times have you said, or heard someone else say, "Today, I'm beginning my new diet. This time, I'll do everything right."

Hey, get real, nobody is perfect here. Yet we set ourselves up for failure by expecting perfection. So how long can you go without "blowing it" and then calling the whole thing off? One week? Three weeks? Three days? Surely some people can last longer than others, yet eventually you begin fantasizing about your favorite unhealthy foods. "Oh, man, all I want is a key lime pie to follow that huge, juicy steak and a monster baked potato dripping with gobs of creamy butter..." and on and on. But no, you think to yourself, "I will be perfect, I will never have another steak again." Yeah, right! And this is how the setup for failure begins...

The Cookie Monster...Not Just a Children's Fantasy Character

If you find yourself really lusting after a cookie or some ice cream *(mint chocolate chip is my personal favorite)*, go to the bakery in the supermarket, buy 2 cookies *(not whole box, which normally has at least 8 to 12 cookies)*, take them home and enjoy. Or go to the frozen yogurt store nearest to you and buy a small or a "kiddie cup" of any kind of non-fat or low-fat frozen yogurt, maybe with a little "fake" hot fudge on top, and then enjoy. When my kids were little, we used to take a weekly Friday afternoon trip to TCBY...Good choice, better control!

The Daily Diet Record and Sample Menu

From 1960 to 2004, the percentage of overweight U.S. adults increased from 44.8 to 66 percent.[3] Today, two thirds of the population is overweight, and pardon me, we are still growing! So obviously, losing weight and keeping it off is not an easy task for most.

Some state that 95 percent of people who lose weight put it back on. I don't believe there are any absolutely reliable, knowledgeable records that know the "real" success rate, but obviously, from the number of weight loss clinics and diet schemes in this country, most people are not successful at keeping off the weight they have lost *(assuming they lose it in the first place)*, no matter in what manner or how much they lost.

Again, and I cannot stress it enough:

YOU MUST CHANGE YOUR HABITS AND BEHAVIORS THAT CAUSED THE WEIGHT GAIN IN THE FIRST PLACE, IN ORDER TO BE SUCCESSFUL AT KEEPING THAT WEIGHT OFF.

The honest awareness of what you have done to gain the weight originally is important for making a permanent change. One of the best ways to change a behavior is to become aware of what your habits are and what prompts you to do those behaviors before you actually do it *(such as where you are, who you are with, how you are feeling)*. If you can train your mind to "think before you act," you then can reestablish a different, more controlled lifestyle.

The Daily Diet Record

By far one of the best methods to accomplish this is to write down what you plan on eating before you eat. This allows you to, at least think about what you are doing, before you do it. You train yourself to take the 20 seconds necessary to ask: "Is this what I really want? Is this worth it? Where will this fat be 'deposited' on me? Will I feel better if I eat this?"

Think about this: A 12-ounce can of regular soda is about 136 calories. The bigger 20-ounce soda in a bottle is about 225 calories! Is it worth all those calories for one lousy soda? Occasionally it is, yet most of the time...NO WAY! So, if you can learn to think about it before you do it and analyze the situation, you are probably going to be less likely to make that poor decision.

Using a daily diet record is, by far, one of the best tools in achieving successful, long-term weight loss. By using this method of documenting your meals ahead of time, you can train your mind and establish new habits and an awareness that help you make better choices while controlling the amount you eat. In my experience, 85 percent of people who are successful at losing weight keep a daily diet record before they eat.

In order to keep the weight off, it is imperative to employ this method for at least one month. This is not something you are committing to doing for the rest of your life, it is just something you should do for a period of time when you first begin the program. After that, you can use your judgment about whether or not or for how long you should continue to use it.

But for at least one month: Each day, write down what you plan to eat before you eat it. You could do it five minutes before, an hour before, or you could be really smart and plan your food menu for a whole week and follow it *(take it with you to the grocery store)*. The results will be fantastic. You are now training your mind to automatically think before you act. What a concept!

Tank McNamara

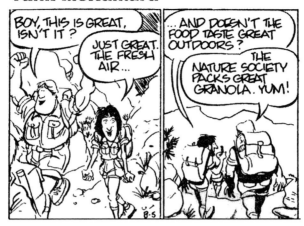

Jeff Millar & Bill Hinds

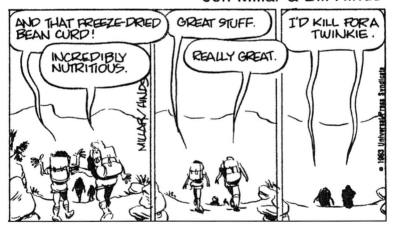

Diet Record

Photocopy and use daily. A small, spiral-bound pad is a handy method too.

Please Copy and Use Weekly.

Food Diary of:

For the Week of:

DAY	DATE	BREAKFAST	BKFAST TIME	LUNCH	LUNCH TIME	SNACK	SNACK TIME	DINNER	DINNER TIME	VITAMINS Y·N	EXERCISE Y·N	COMMENTS, PROBLEMS & FEELINGS
SUN												
MON												
TUE												
WED												
THU												
FRI												
SAT												

Three Day Sample Menu

Day 1

Breakfast:	2 slices whole-wheat toast *(not diet bread)*
	1 oz. low-fat cheese
	1 fruit
Lunch:	1 bowl *(two cups)* of "hearty soup" *(minestrone, lentil, tomato & rice)*
	1/2 sandwich *(1 oz. low-fat meat, i.e. chicken, tuna, turkey, mustard, lettuce & tomato)*
Afternoon snack:	1 cereal bar, 140 calories *(ex. NutriGrain, Kashi)*
Supper:	3-4 oz. low-fat meat
	3/4 cup of any starch *(rice, potato, corn, peas, beans)*
	Any amount of broccoli, other greens or salad
	(30 calories per Tbsp. salad dressing)
Evening treat:	3 cups popcorn or one low-fat ice cream bar

Day 2

Breakfast:	6 oz vanilla Dannon Low Fat Yogurt on top of 3/4 cup of cereal *(fiber type)*
	1/2 large banana on top of yogurt and cereal

Lunch:	6" Subway Veggie Delight on a whole-wheat sub roll with All the veggie trimmings with either mustard or light on the mayo
Afternoon snack:	1 cereal bar, different flavor, or small bag of baked Lays Potato Chips
Supper:	"Meatless Supper"
	¾ cup brown rice *(use soy sauce)*
	¾ cup Lima or black beans *(add salsa)*
	Add vegetable or chicken bouillon to rice/beans while cooking *(canned beans are OK)*
	Mixed green salad, low fat-dressing. Enjoy.
Evening treat:	1 Popsicle *(for example, Dole, Weight Watchers)*

Day 3

Breakfast:	1 whole bagel *(preferably whole wheat or oat bran)*
	1 Tbsp. light cream cheese
	1 fruit
Lunch:	Veggie Burger *(Garden Burger or Boca Burger)* on bun or wheat bread with Condiments: lite mayo, ketchup, mustard
	1 dill pickle
	Option: If necessary, 1 small bag Baked Lays Potato Chips
Afternoon snack:	3 cups popcorn or 1 slice wheat bread with jam

Supper:	1 frozen meal *(Amy's, Health Choice, Lean Cuisine, Kashi)*
	Large mixed salad *(water chestnuts add crunch)* with lite dressing
Evening treat:	2/3 cup frozen yogurt or lite ice cream

Fluids During Meals

Suggested beverage choices during mealtime are: water, water, water, unsweetened or lightly sweetened tea, water, diet soda *(if need be)*. Try sparkling water for variety, particularly with the large bubbles. It's delightful. The smaller bubbles seem to "fizz" more. A few brand names to try *(with the larger bubbles)* are: La Croix, Ritz, and Syfo. There are too many brands to mention, but some old stand-bys are Perrier, Voss or San Pellegrino. If out to eat, you can also just ask for soda water from the bar.

A Note on Water and Fiber: For fiber to do an adequate sweeping and sponging job in your digestive tract, there has to be an adequate amount of water in the system for it to absorb. Otherwise, fiber may actually contribute to constipation rather than prevent it, or it may soak up water and other nutrients needed elsewhere by the body. Fiber does a world of good for your body, so help it do its job by drinking plenty of water. **See more on water, in the chapter "Vitamins, Minerals and Water."

Attitude and Awareness

Motivation: Some Have It, Some Don't

"You don't want to become comfortable being uncomfortable with yourself," stated one of my more introspective clients.

Over the years, I have learned a lot about the trials and tribulations of weight loss from my clients of a variety of ages, income levels, racial/ethnic groups, and cultural backgrounds. If you are reading this book, chances are that you have decided that (a) you do not have to give up and accept your situation and (b) you want to finally do this *(lose weight)* the right way.

Let's look at the reality of the situation:

TRUTH

DESIRE

FAITH

WORK

Consider saying these words, either out-loud or to yourself:
The TRUTH is I am overweight.
I DESIRE to not be overweight.

I have the FAITH that I can change my lifestyle and habits.
Yet, I must WORK at a daily routine to achieve this goal.

Part of the problem, of course, is the work. However, for the most part you know that anything positive you have ever achieved in your life did not "just happen" to you. You had to work at it, get better at it, and make it happen. When you did this, it became yours. You earned the right to be rewarded.

It is truly the same with permanent weight control. If you work at following this Path that I am laying out for you, you will become normal weight. And you will not only become normal weight, you will also be leading a healthier lifestyle and decreasing your chances of getting a number of diseases.

Concepts to Help You Stay Motivated
(and not get too frustrated along the way!)

Concept One: How often should I weigh?

Glad you asked! Some people weigh themselves daily, same time, same place, ritualistically. Some folks head straight for the grocery store in the morning...don't even eat breakfast...just so they can get on the store's scale before heading to work. Some folks weigh both morning and night. These obsessive tactics are not good!

I realize that it can be difficult to not become obsessed with the scale, but please realize that becoming obsessed with the scale is self-defeating and does not make sense. Your weight fluctuates slightly throughout the day, depending on many factors. I suggest WEIGHING ONCE A WEEK, at the same time, using the same scale, and wearing same amount of clothing/shoes (*or lack of*). Do not focus on the scale during the rest of the week. Instead, focus on the habits, behaviors and routine that I have suggested.

Concept Two: Lose one and a half pounds per week.

There is an old joke that everyone wants to lose 30 pounds by Friday. Obviously, that is ridiculous and unrealistic. So how much should you expect to lose on a consistent basis? I have found that for many clients *(but not all)*, losing an average of 1 1/2 pounds per week is realistic and attainable. You may say that that is not enough, "In the past, I've lost 3 pounds a week." Or "Susan, in my office, is losing 2 and 3 pounds per week!" But if you really focus on the habits and behaviors and consistently average 1 1/2 pounds weekly, that will become six pounds per month and 72 pounds per year! Now do you see where I'm going with this? *(This is assuming that you actually have that much to lose...some do, some don't.)* One and a half pounds per week is obviously a very good goal to reach. Remember that the faster you lose weight, the more likely you are to put it back on...IF a lifestyle change does not go along with it.

Concept Three: Patterns of Weight Loss

Often people expect to lose weight weekly, then a week or two goes by when it doesn't happen, and they say, "Forget it, I quit!" Over the years, I have realized that this is part of an interesting but uncommonly discussed phenomenon that I call "The Patterns of Weight Loss."

Some people will lose the same amount of weight consistently each week. Some will lose or drop pounds every two weeks, or even in three or four week segments. Talk about frustration! Why is this? I have consulted people such as Dr. Kelly Brownell, obesity research expert, currently at Yale University and previously at the University of Pennsylvania. He too saw this aberrant pattern. "We have seen this as well in our Obesity Research Institute at the University of Pennsylvania School Of

Medicine," he told me.

Examine your own situation when you find yourself experiencing these fluctuating patterns. Did your eating routine change in any way? Did you really stick with the plan? Regardless of how you answer these questions, realize that there are some people who are very focused and follow the plan to the letter and still do not lose pounds on a weekly basis! There may be reasons for that. Record your weekly weigh-ins, make a chart or log, and realize that although you may not lose weekly, if you are doing the right thing, a pattern of weight loss will in fact be established.

Concept Four: The Set Point or "Plateau"

How many times have you dieted, lost some weight and then completely stopped losing? You were "stuck." When the scale wouldn't budge, panic set in.

Your rational mind may have recognized that you were hitting a plateau, but your emotional mind was probably, to put it bluntly, "pissed off." Now what to do about it? Starve yourself? Plunge into a large ice cream cone and admit defeat? No!

A plateau is a weight level that your body has known previously, maybe last year, two years ago, or longer. For example: You are 5'3" and 142 pounds. You come head-to-head with some major relationship issues, life becomes unusually frustrating, and you begin eating anything available. You gain weight. At 158 pounds, you're still consuming too much food, but your weight stays steady. You realize that, a few years ago, you were also at this weight for some length of time. Normally, you should still be gaining, but you are not. This is a plateau on the upswing.

A plateau also can occur in the downward direction. You are doing great, staying on your weight loss plan, and have lost 12 pounds from the 170 pounds you started at. You hit the historic 158 pounds and then can not drop anymore pounds. Aha! That old plateau has hit, also known as a set point. In 1982, authors William Bennett, MD and Joel Gurin informed us of this discouraging phenomenon in their book, "The Dieter's Dilemma: Eating Less and Weighing More."

So great, now what do I do? There is hope. To break the plateau, or set point, you must either further decrease calories or increase exercise. In order to work through this plateau *(without starving yourself)*, simply recognize that you have been stuck there before and continue, steadfast, on your new regime.

Concept Five: Increments of 10

How many times have you thought about losing weight and yet, were daunted by how much weight you needed to lose? How often has the task seemed too great, leaving you feeling hopeless?

Some people make a plan in the beginning about how much they need to lose and how long it will take. The thought can, in some cases, quickly become overwhelming. "So why bother?" you may think.

Let's start this thought process over. THINK ABOUT THE POUNDS YOU NEED TO LOSE IN INCREMENTS OF 10.

Say you weigh 282 pounds. You are 5'6" and realistically, you would like to weigh 140 pounds. "My God, I need to lose 142 pounds!" you think in disbelief. Yes, anyone would find that extremely overwhelming and would probably become discouraged before even making an attempt.

Instead, here is how you should think: "I will focus on the '10's.' I am currently 282, so my focus, my goal, will be to 'Say goodbye to the 280's and hello to the 270's!' Once I reach that goal, I will be proud of myself and feel a sense of accomplishment. Then, I will set a new goal and begin working toward it. I will work through the 270's, until I can say 'Hello 260's!' I will be proud of and praise myself with each goal reached."

In increments of 10, you will eventually reach your ultimate goal, and you will do so with much less frustration and more positive regard for yourself.

Concept Six: Satisfied vs. Full vs. Stuffed

Obviously, *(if you are willing to admit it)* you eat too much! Epiphany! So, how do I know when to stop? Part of the problem is taking the correct food portion sizes in the first place. We just don't know when "enough is enough." Earlier, I mentioned using the "Freddy Plate," a smaller, salad-size plate instead of the normally large dinner plate. This really does help you eat less, because you initially have less space to pile on the food *(and yet you still get the satisfaction of sitting down to eat with a full plate of food)*. While eating a meal, how many times have you all of a sudden realized, "Oh, man...I've eaten too much!" Many times, I'm sure. Consider portions and ponder the "State of the Stomach." It does have its boundaries, just like any other state, and you must be aware not to push those boundaries. They are there for a reason.

Feeling Satisfied:

Eating until you are satisfied involves eating slowly, with a finite amount of food available, then stopping and doing something else. Being satisfied is a feeling that you want to tune in to. Feeling happy and content with yourself is wonderful. Yes, you could eat more *(we all could eat more, all the time)*. FEELING SATISFIED IS NOT THE SAME THING AS FEELING LIKE YOU

SIMPLY CAN'T EAT ANYMORE. When you are satisfied (*often you have stopped eating*), you should be able to: sit in a movie comfortably, walk down the street for 10 minutes without feeling sick, or even maybe (*PG-13 warning!*) have sex after a meal. You typically cannot do these things very well if you are full.

Feeling Full:

Eating until you are full is when you get up from the table and ask yourself, "Why did I do that?" Now, you are uncomfortable. "Maybe I'll loosen my belt a bit or undo the first button of my pants," you think to yourself. If only you had stopped a little sooner, you would have been just fine and would not have had to resort to the covert "under the table unbuttoning" move. You filled yourself up to the brim and lacked restraint. Now you are feeling a little guilty and making excuses for why you ate more than you needed to. Note: If you have gotten used to eating until you feel full, you may have "forgotten" the difference between feeling full and feeling satisfied, and you may need to deliberately train yourself to become more aware of and recognize this difference. Ask yourself, "Is this something I need to work on?"

Feeling Stuffed:

We all know this feeling - it is not a good one. The revulsion or disgust caused by overindulgence or excess can be overwhelming. For some of us, this primarily happens on Thanksgiving...which is accepted, allowed, desired, expected and just down right OK! What cruel soul would intentionally insult Grandma anyway, know what I mean?

Stuffed is where you can barely get up from the table, you put your eye on the sofa, and oh so carefully, mosey your way to the couch. Of course, the problem is that this happens all too frequently when it's not Thanksgiving, right? For many, it is a daily routine.

Not many of my clients who weigh more than 250 pounds would admit it *(some, just because they do not realize it)*, but they often feel they must eat until they are hurting or stuffed. In fact, this becomes the norm, the routine, and the expected. They think: "A meal is not complete until I experience feeling stuffed." Then afterward, talk about misgivings: "I wish I hadn't, but I did." "Oh well, won't do that again!" But they keep doing it. Of course, this isn't limited to the dining table. This may lead to excess or overindulgence elsewhere, as well. Regardless of whether this mentality was learned in your adult life or childhood, regardless of if it is cultural, if your parents grew up during the Great Depression, or if your family had little money and thus, you learned as a child to eat as much food as possible when it was available, you need to leave this habit behind. Aside from Thanksgiving, you should do everything in your power to prevent yourself from becoming "stuffed."

Concept Seven: The First Three Bites

Which tastes better, the first three bites or the last three bites? *("All of it!" is not an answer choice.)* I ask this to many people, and they admittedly answer, "The first three bites." Think about it.

So taste is certainly not the only reason that we continuously overeat. Why DO we continue to fill our mouths long after we have felt the initial satisfaction?

1. It is in front of us.

2. We belong to "The Clean Plate Club" and think, "I am not finished eating until my plate is clean, regardless of how full I may feel."

3. We are thinking of the starving children in _____ *(China?*

Somalia? Just fill in the blank).

4. I paid for it!

Think about this: You are at your local frozen yogurt or ice cream shop, ready to order. The attendant behind the counter offers you small, medium, large, or "grande." You are thinking, "The small is too small, the medium is okay...but I'm a little hungry. Besides that, I haven't been bad for at least 24 hours *(Ha!)*, so I might as well have the large." Halfway through the large, you somehow realize *(because of that instinctual, uncomfortable feeling that you would like to ignore)* that you have had enough. But you still have another 5 ounces, so what the heck, you keep eating until there is nothing left in the bowl, even though you had really already reached satisfaction.

You knew that the first three bites were the best, but you are in the habit of finishing what is in front of you, so the rest is history. If you had ordered the small size and eaten it slowly, I bet you would still realize halfway through that you had already enjoyed the best part. So start with less, eat as slowly as possible, and you will gain that feeling of satisfaction not long after that first few bites of your favorite flavor of cold frozen yogurt or low-fat ice cream hits your tongue.

Positive Intelligent Thinking:
Revelations of the Mind

The mind controls all *(or at least most)* of what we do. Often, revelations concerning the mind over food are apparent. My clients' difficulties with food have taught me, as mentioned:

YOU DON'T WANT TO BE COMFORTABLE BEING UNCOMFORTABLE WITH YOURSELF.

Say you weigh 303 pounds, you are 6 feet tall, and you have been carrying around this bulk for 15 years. You lost 30 pounds and then gained back 40, then lost some more and regained it again. After a while, you become "comfortable" with yourself at this size. Except your knees are "killing you" and your newly diagnosed type 2 diabetes may really kill you... But you are accepting yourself as you are, while your body slowly heads toward obesity. Not a good place to be. There must be another way.

Anesthetizing the Mind with Food

Often, we want to turn off our brain for so many reasons. To quote a client: "Reality sucks!" so he eats. He thinks, "Whatever is going wrong...whatever hits the fan...if I eat, at least while I'm eating, I won't be concerned with my problems."

It could be anything. Your boss wants more work from you; your spouse adds to the "honey do" list; your kids at college want more money; your own health is deteriorating. So what is the easiest and quickest escape? Eating, of course! While eating, the mind is on hold and the mouth, tongue, and pleasure senses are engaged, so all is right with the world... for the moment.

Temptation and Greed

"I want it. I want it now. I want all of it. I want it for as long as I want. I don't want limitations. I don't want to be told how much I can eat or when I should eat."

The sad situation is no matter how much we have, it never feels like enough. We always want more. We are enticed by the promise of pleasure or gain to excessively buy things we really don't need. We don't need every new technological "gizmo" on the market. We don't need a different pair of shoes for every outfit or every day of the week.

The "Emotional Rescue"
(not just a Rolling Stones song)

The above-referenced song talks about "coming to your emotional rescue." Although Mick Jaggar may have been talking about a love interest, many of us turn to food as our emotional rescue, also known as "Emotional Eating."

"My boss is annoyed with me. My partner is mad at me. My kids won't listen. My life is frustrating. I need something to eat!" Many of us feel that way. The problem is: if we act on that feeling too often, it becomes the common and over-used easy answer of the moment. "If I could just have a piece of key lime pie, I could feel better." And very likely you will, from the moment the sweet tanginess hits your tongue until the moment it leaves. Then, the guilt will hit, and you will probably wind up feeling worse than you did before you ate the pie. Drats!

Instead of eating, do something else. Do something positive, less damaging and even emotionally satisfying! For example, instead of putting food in your mouth, go call a friend, take a short walk, pick up a magazine, take a hot shower/bath, wash your car, go to the movies or finish a project. You don't want to do it, but once you clean that room, you really will feel better about it! Are you really hungry? Is it your stomach or is it your emotions growling? You will experience a deeper, longer-lasting feeling of happiness from completing a task than from eating a piece of pie. *(Yes, even key lime pie.)*

Give Me a Kiss…Hershey or Otherwise!

Where did you go the last time you felt rejected, lonely or unloved? Did you go to the kitchen to check out the refrigerator…just to make sure everything was still there? Or did you leave the house and head to the supermarket because there was something you really wanted, although you weren't quite sure what?

It's 9:15 p.m. You enter the store and begin to "cruise" the aisles. What do you want? Is it bread, sweets, ice cream, or maybe, just maybe, chocolate? Eventually, you somehow find yourself in the chocolate section. There are almond bars, peanut butter cups and even high quality Swiss chocolate (*dark, semisweet, milk, raspberry filling, hazelnut…*), luscious to the palate, and euphoric to the brain….you want some.

Now, imagine that there happens to be a thoroughly attractive individual standing nearby, eyeing the same shelf of chocolate. She/He asks you which brand is the best. As your eyes meet, (*maybe*) you suddenly realize that what you are longing for is not really the cocoa. You are there for your emotional hunger. You crave interesting or exciting conversation, kindness, someone caring about your opinion, or someone to gaze back into your eyes and say, "I love you."

All the while your desire for chocolate wanes and mild infatuation begins. You are feeling good, and you haven't even consumed any calories! What is happening here? We must separate feelings from food. Food is not love. We may love food, but it does not love us back (*and we stop loving it once it reaches our waist*). We need food to live, but we can live a happier life with love. This love can and will hopefully be in the form of meaningful relationships – not necessarily romantic - it could be familial or close friendship as well. We also need a love of life. There are many things we can do in life that can bring us joy and be fulfilling *(without adding unnecessary calories)*.

Now, let's talk about the Hershey Kiss. Throughout my experience of nutritional counseling, the most universal food people desire is chocolate. Not everybody, but many. You may have heard of a chemical compound called phenylethylamine. It seems when people are either in love or infatuated, the brain kicks-up production of this substance.

When people are victims of unrequited love or fall out of love, they may go through a type of mild depression in which the brain irregularly produces this substance. Therefore, they often binge on chocolate during their periods of depression. So why chocolate? Researchers have shown that chocolate contains substantial amounts of phenylethylamine. Therefore, the chocolate cravings come when this substance is low or lacking. Knowing this, you can reduce the chocolate calories by "reaching for your mate instead of your plate." *(Or if you don't have a mate, some good laughs with friends will make you feel better because of increased endorphin production.)*

Haven't you ever wondered why chocolate is so popular on Valentine's Day? Nothing like a double dose of phenylethylamine, also known as a "lover's high!"

It is believed to work by making the brain release b-endorphin, an opioid peptide which is the driving force behind the pleasurable effects. That's the good news. The bad news is that most chocolate contains a lot of fat and a lot of sugar, yet only a little cocoa *(where the phenylethylamine actually comes from)*. From *Food Values of Portions Commonly Used*, by Dr. Jean Pennington, the breakdown of chocolate is: 60-70% fat, 20-30% sugar, and 4-6% cocoa. Exotic or imported semi-sweet or dark chocolate is usually significantly better and may contain 20-25% pure chocolate *(compared to the 4-6% in milk chocolate)*. And for the true connoisseurs, bittersweet chocolate is 35% pure.[4] Other lesser known facts about chocolate: It contains only 1/10th the amount of caffeine as a cup of brewed coffee!

Additionally, research by Dr. Scott Grundy and Dr. Margo Denke, from the University of Texas' Southwestern Medical Center, has shown to the surprise of many that the saturated fat found in chocolate is not the same kind of fat that is found in butter, lard or milk. They discovered that the principal fatty acid in cocoa butter, stearic acid, actually does not raise your cholesterol level to the same degree as other types of saturated fats.[5]

So, should you combine the following, touted good for you "sins" – a bar of chocolate, a glass of red wine, and a spoonful of olive oil – to lower your cholesterol levels? As my Victorian grandmother who lived to be 97 used to say, "Moderation, babe!"

What about the calories? We all know that chocolate contains a lot of calories. Each Hershey Kiss contains 25 calories, while a Three Musketeers Bar contains 280 calories! So how about four Hershey Kisses to satisfy the sweet tooth instead of a whole candy bar?

Chocolate seems to have a close relative in peanut butter. The nutritional breakdown is: 60-80% fat, 10-20% sugar and 10-15% protein. So chocolate and peanut butter are similar. As a teenager, my son, who considered himself an expert on chocolate, termed peanut butter, "The Healthy Chocolate." Some taste trials have shown people reporting the taste of peanut butter as an acceptable alternative to chocolate. How often do you reach for the peanut butter jar when you are too lazy to drive to the store for a chocolate fix?

Think about it. What do you find on your pillow at night when you and your sweetie are at that romantic bed and breakfast? Chocolate is really a mood elevator and is known as the "love drug." Next time you get that craving, stop and think about it, and try satisfying that need through interacting with a person. You never know who you may meet at the grocery store...even at 3 a.m., while looking for Mr. Goodbar *(the chocolate one, that is)*.

When It Feels Good To Be Bad

You have completed your work. You called your mother and listened to her problems, as you dutifully do daily. You are such a perfect person. But now it is time to be bad! When you're bad, it's because you deserve it. It is your reward. **News flash!** You are not perfect, nor do you have to be. This brings us back to the earlier concept of "Staying on the program or staying with the program. When you are on it and doing well, great, but then you blow it...you go to Aunt Martha's and consume her world famous chocolate cake with ice cream on the side. Who wouldn't?! OK, so next meal, next day, get back on the program. It isn't all or nothing. Nobody is perfect. Don't beat up on yourself; just get back on the program.

Eating wisely is a long-term endeavor with short-term failures/experiences but results in long-term success.

A Sweet for My Sweetie

We eat too much sugar, in all forms: cakes, candies, pies, sodas, even cereals. In fact, according to the USDA, Americans consume an average of 152 pounds of caloric sweeteners in one year![6] One

Beetle Bailey

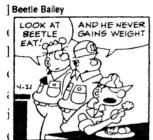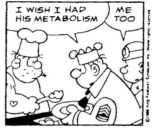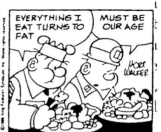

Reprinted with special permission of King Features Syndicate, Inc.

Take a look at the approximate number of teaspoons of sugar in these food items:

	Teaspoons
1 slice cake, iced	**12**
12 ounce soda pop	**9**
1 slice pie	**9**
1/2 cup sherbet	**6**
1 glazed donut	**6**
1 cup flavored yogurt	**6**
1/2 cup ice cream	**3**
1 ice cream cone	**3**
2 small cookies	**3**
1/2 cup canned fruit (light syrup)	**3**
1/2 cup sweetened cereal	**3**
1 candy bar	**3**

Food Addictions and Cravings

Many people I meet in my practice complain that they are addicted to certain foods, most often a starch or carbohydrate. The rise and fall of your blood sugar controls your hunger and your desire to eat. So if you wait too long to eat or are not timely with your meals, you will create an "addiction" or craving for whatever will make you feel better and certainly, whatever raises and sustains your blood sugar will satisfy that craving.

Simple sugars *(sweets or foods with added sugar)* satisfy your cravings almost immediately, but they do not "stay with you" *(sustain you)* for long. So instead, stick with complex carbohydrates or starches, such as whole grain products *(brown rice, whole grain cereal/pasta/bread, etc.)*, which both satisfy the appetite for longer and sustain the blood sugar.

"Snacking" is Not a Dirty Word

"Snacking" has a negative connotation to it, especially for those trying to lose weight. The problem with snacking comes from the fact that when we do it, we are often not "in control" of our habits, and we therefore make poor choices about what or what amount. Snacking "because I feel like it," because you are bored, or because of emotional reasons *(instead of because you are hungry)* is not a good decision. But there really is nothing wrong with snacking, IF it is done at the right time, with the right snack, and in reasonable amounts. In fact, for most of us, we would be better off eating five or six small meals each day, instead of two or three larger ones. Yet, in the normal school or work day, eating every few hours is often not realistic. So an alternative is to routinely eat the right starches and whole grains, in order to sustain the blood sugar and keep the hunger at bay for longer.

Of course, most of us love to snack. Sometimes it's a feeling of "getting away with something" that we think we should not do. Other times, we are overcome by an absolute urge to snack. This could be for a lot of different reasons. Here are some scenarios:

The "At Work" Snack

It is 4 p.m., and you need a break from reality. You leave your office in a daze from the work day. Your legs automatically take you "where you need to go." You find yourself down the hall, staring point-blank at the snack machine and its kaleidoscope of choices.

Of course, for some of us, there is no need for choices, because we always get the same "yummy" treat, say a Snickers bar. For others, the problem IS choice. Oh, the choices! The conscience steps in, and the choice is between a healthier, lower calorie snack *(maybe pretzels, popcorn, a granola bar, or better yet, the apple you brought from home)* or a "The Devil Made Me Do It!" type of choice. Are you stronger than the Devil? Usually not!

For a working person, the 3 to 4 p.m. snack is that "break from reality" or reward for a hard day's work, so planning is essential. Of course, if you don't pre-plan to bring a healthy alternative to work, then you are at the mercy of the all-powerful snack machine. Pack healthy snacks that provide some sustenance, such as a cereal bar, an apple, a small bag of low-fat microwave popcorn *(did you know that popcorn is a whole-grain food?)*, or for some variety, a healthy trail mix. To save money and to decrease sugar content, you can make your own trail mix at home by filling a small baggie with raisins or other dried fruit, broken pretzels, popcorn, cereal, and nuts. When choosing dried fruit, try to find some with no sugar added *(sometimes hard to do if not at a health food store)* or play it safe with raisins. If you are the type of "snacker" who tends to snack not because you are hungry but simply because of the need to chew or suck on something, Tootsie Roll pops, a small box of raisins, a small bag of grapes *(ever tried them frozen?)* or a crunchy lightly-sweetened whole-grain cereal *(like Frosted Mini-Wheats, Kashi Go-Lean Crunch or Honey-Nut Cheerios)* may curb your need. Just eat each piece slowly, for more satisfaction.

Sometimes, we even mistake thirst for the need for food in our mouth. A cold glass of water or low-sugar drink *(try a cold glass of water with a splash of juice)* may also help satisfy this need. It is a good idea to have a glass or bottle of water with you at all times.

There is nothing wrong with a well-planned afternoon snack break. An unplanned and unhealthy snack break, on the other hand, can have further reaching effects than just that one poor choice. Guilt may creep in and you might say, "What the heck, I might as well have fried chicken for supper since I already blew it once today." This is the beginning of the downward spiral of unhealthy eating patterns.

The Evening Snack

This is another common pitfall. The evening snack raises its ugly head any time between supper and bedtime. Maybe you begin snacking immediately after supper, even if you are not still hungry. Or maybe come early evening, you settle in for a little TV watching. Then, when the first food commercial comes on, you levitate from your easy chair into the kitchen to survey the snack possibilities. Don't fool yourself...children are not the only ones that the media affects!

Some people, me included, wait until bedtime and have a snack in bed just before "lights out." There is even the middle of the night "I can't sleep" snack which is the most dangerous because nobody is awake to see you, and you may feel that you can eat as much as you want. You get sleepy *(i.e. full again)* and will probably have forgotten about it by morning, so you tend to forget that guilt. Can we talk?!

The Evening Snack - Revisited

You are now midway between supper and bedtime. Normally, you have a snack while watching the tube or using the computer.

Sometimes the best time to enjoy and control a small evening snack is right before bedtime, not in the middle of the evening while in front of the television. *(THAT'S DANGEROUS! Even worse is in the kitchen after supper.)* Best suggestion for a late evening snack, a popsicle or 3/4 cup of your favorite low-fat frozen yogurt or sorbet *(Ben & Jerry's and Hagen Daas have some options, among other brands)*, **in bed**, right before bedtime. Bring in the world's smallest spoon *(helps you eat slower)* and maybe turn on the tube or enjoy a book, magazine or newspaper, and relax *(see snack list)*. Remember to savor the flavor! Sweet and satisfying, but not something you will have to spend half of the next day on a treadmill to burn off. Get up and brush your teeth! Change the flavor in your mouth quickly, and you will be less likely to desire more. Food never seems as appetizing when you have that "minty fresh" feeling in your mouth!

REMEMBER: WHATEVER YOU DO:
DO NOT GO BACK INTO THE KITCHEN!
THAT IS DANGEROUS TERRITORY!

For some people, just having a low-calorie, warm, sweet beverage while watching television is sufficient. The International Flavored Coffees or a cup of steamy hot chocolate *(or cold chocolate milk if it's summer)* does the trick. Now you've enjoyed your late evening snack... Get out of bed, wash the cup in the bathroom sink and leave it there. Brush and floss your teeth, and go back to bed. Do not go back to the kitchen tonight! There is no need to!

The After-School Snack

For many children *(or high school or college students)*, the afternoon snack – right after school - is the first snack of the day. The child arrives home, heads to the kitchen, surveys the bounty and begins putting a variety of snacks on the counter. Of course, this is not true of all kids. But if you have a teen or child who is overweight or at-risk for becoming overweight, it is more likely that this does occur. Most kids have a snack after school. There is nothing wrong with that. The key is to have the right low-fat foods available so that when they grab "whatever's there," the "whatever's there" is not something you feel guilty allowing your child to put in his/her body.

If your kitchen pantry and refrigerator are stocked with primarily low-fat choices and just a few high fat options *(deemed as "dessert only" items, preferably in a out-of-site cabinet)*, everyone is better off. Later in the book, I have a selection of these, such as low-calorie popsicles, popcorn and pretzels. Remember that it is not fair to keep lots of unhealthy options in the kitchen and then expect your child to have the self-discipline to stay away from them *(you know how hard it is for you...it is probably twice as hard for them)*. Likewise, it is not fair to have unhealthy foods that the adults are allowed to eat but the kids are not.

The "Arriving Home After-Work" Snack

This is always challenging. Which is the first room you enter in your house upon arriving home from work? For many, it is the kitchen. The side door or garage usually leads us right there. Many may have no clue where our front door is because we haven't used it in years.

One reasonable, quick solution to controlling snacking is to enter through the front door and go directly to your bedroom.

No, I am not advocating to "sleep off" the craving! Change your clothes – put on your "around the house, comfortable stuff" – then brush your teeth for a new, clean taste in your mouth.

Then, go get the mail. Now, if you need something to hold you over until dinner, go into the kitchen and plan your snack. The idea is to change snacking from an impulsive behavior into a well thought-out one. By changing the habit of heading immediately for the kitchen, you give yourself time to figure out, "Am I snacking because it is a habit? Or am I snacking because I really am hungry and need something to hold me over?" This way, you also give yourself time to figure out what to eat.

Find a low-fat, satisfying treat. Even if you take out your favorite crackers and peanut butter, have a plan. For instance, place four crackers with a reasonable amount of peanut butter *("dust" it on...no "plopping!")* on a plate. Then, put away the box of crackers and the jar of peanut butter. Get them out of sight! Next, pour yourself a glass of water / diet soda / light tea and take the plate of goodies out of the kitchen. Sit down and slowly enjoy your snack *(maybe while you are trying to think of what to do for dinner).* When you are finished, put your empty plate and glass in the sink *(you'll wash them later),* and leave the kitchen. Get out of the kitchen. Be gone from the kitchen! Got it?!

You have probably heard of this suggested remedy for difficulty falling asleep: Use your bedroom only for sleeping *(or other intimate activities)* and not for anything else. The same idea applies for trying to break the habit of impulsive eating. Only spend time in your kitchen when you are cooking or eating. Don't go in there otherwise. Do not "hang out" in the kitchen too long *(for some that may mean more than two minutes and you are bound to start eating).* It is the power of association.

The "It's the Weekend and I Can Do Whatever I Want" Snack

Definitely the most likely open-ended snacking situation is the weekend. You sleep late on Saturday morning, skip breakfast, move slowly, have no schedule, and extend your morning coffee time with the newspaper and lounging. On the weekend, it is certainly necessary to relax, but it is not necessary to completely forget about your routine. Even if you sleep in, be sure to still have breakfast soon after you arise.

Then, try to get back in-synch by having lunch closer to the time when you usually eat. This way, you are not snacking throughout the day because your blood sugar is dropping and your body doesn't know what is going on.

Also, in preventing unnecessary weekend eating, it is helpful to have a general plan for your weekend day. Do something fun or get something done that you need to do. Go to garage sales, the movies, a book store, or garden nurseries. Take a walk with a friend, partner, or family member in a park (*if you like the outdoors*) or downtown (*if you are more the window-shopping type*). There is plenty you can do to entertain yourself by spending little or no money and even better, while moving. Take care of your "Honey-Do" list. Get some outside exercise. Don't waste your day hanging out at home, glued to the tube, asking yourself "What can I eat?"

Remember, snacking is not a dirty word. It can actually be used as a tool to help you reach your weight loss goals. However, you must hold your snacking decisions to the same standard as your meal decisions. You also must have healthy snack foods available to you whenever possible (*which is mostly dependent on your grocery shopping trips*). Change your perspective of snacking from an impulsive, habitual behavior to a behavior that serves a purpose (*such as curbing your hunger or buying you time before your next meal)* and that does so in a healthy way. Healthy snacking can actually put you closer to your weight loss and healthy lifestyle goals, as opposed to putting you further behind. For the next week, concentrate on changing the way you think about snacking. Redefine the word in your mind, and remember this during your next trip to the grocery store.

Disease States You Don't Want

The Why's of Today's Modern Health Problems

You name it, we've got it: type 2 diabetes *(also known as adult-onset diabetes)*, heart disease, breast cancer, prostate cancer, gastric reflux, colon/rectal cancer, hypertension *(high blood pressure)*, poor circulation, limited mobility, indigestion, elevated lipid *(fat)* levels, breathing disorders, leg ulcers, back pain, knee pain and the ever present obesity. Just wonderful! Have we ever got problems!

These are predominately problems that we could avoid or make ourselves less likely to get. Our present lifestyles are largely contributing to these problems. Do not let me hear you say, "Oh, I'm getting old. At age 38, I have to accept these health problems." Of course not! Get a grip!

Many of these problems are related to weight, undeniably! But we often say things such as: "Oh, I have high sugar and my momma also had high sugar, so it runs in the family." But, maybe your momma also weighed 285 pounds...and she wasn't 7 feet tall either *(nothing against your mom, by the way)*! Yes, genetics are part of the problem...but they are certainly not the WHOLE problem.

123

How Long Do You Want To Live?

What a question! How long do you want to live? What would you like to die from? How do you want your quality of life to be before you die? "Gee, thanks for asking," you say.

Carrying excess body weight can increase your risk of developing or worsening nearly any existing medical condition, such as diabetes, heart disease, stroke, hypertension *(high blood pressure)*, sleep apnea and osteoarthritis.

Twenty years ago, nutrition scientists used large or obese-bred mice in a unique experiment. The scientists gave the "naturally big-boned" mice as much food as they could eat. They then observed them to see how long they lived and what diseases *(diabetes, heart disease, cancer)* they died from.

Next, the scientists created a second group of the same strain of mice and gave them HALF the number of calories as the original group. The result: The second group lived twice as long as the first group and did not frequently die from the diseases suffered by the first group. Take home message: The two groups of mice had the same genetic makeup; the only difference between them was the amount of food they ate. More recently this same study was repeated with similar results.

Evidently, being overweight or obese plays a large role in the longevity of mice. Could it be the same for humans? Think about it. Recently, another study looked at morbidity and mortality tables. Researchers specifically looked at tables that noted heights and weights of men at their time of death. The researchers also discarded those who died of diseases such as AIDS and some forms of cancer. The findings were eye-opening, especially for Americans.

The men who lived the longest who were: 6'2" in height and weighed 175 to 185 pounds. Those at 5'9" in height weighed 150 to 160 pounds. At 5'7" in height, they weighed 145-155 pounds. And all were non-smokers.

What this study revealed is that by being lighter in weight, eating fewer calories and having less total fat in your diet, you do not overwork your vital organs.

Onto the lifestyle-related diseases *(the diseases that you can actually decrease your risk of getting or make less severe if you already have them)*...

Type 2 Diabetes

Type 2 diabetes *(adult-onset diabetes)* has a proven genetic component, but other factors such as an unhealthy diet, a sedentary lifestyle and obesity have caused an epidemic of this disease in America.

First Let's Define Type 1 and Type 2 Diabetes

In Type 1 diabetes *(formerly called "juvenile" or "insulin-dependent" diabetes)* the body has little or no insulin because the immune system – which normally fights off harmful bacteria or viruses – has attacked and destroyed the insulin-producing cells in the pancreas, a gland just behind the stomach.

Type 2 diabetes *(formerly called "adult-onset" or "non insulin-dependent" diabetes)* is a disease in which blood glucose levels are above normal. With this type of diabetes, people have problems converting food to energy and the glucose in the blood increases while the cells are starved of energy.

When you eat, particularly when you eat starches *(rice, noodles, sweet potatoes, cereal, bread, beans, peas (not green English peas) or lentils)* your pancreas releases insulin. The purpose of insulin is to transport this starch *(which has now become glycogen or sugar)* out of the blood stream, across the cell membrane *(wall surrounding each cell)*, and into the cell, where it produces energy for your body. Got it? You need insulin available to convert that starch into energy.

Here is the problem. If body fat is surrounding the cell, the body fat will prevent the sugar from entering the cell. In this case, the insulin will instead, deposit the sugar into the bloodstream, which raises your blood sugar. And eventually, if your blood sugar gets too high, you may be told by your physician that you have diabetes, specifically type 2 diabetes. Type 2 diabetes constitutes about 85% to 95% of all diabetes cases in developed countries and accounts for an even higher percentage in developing countries.[7]

Obesity is a major factor in the development of insulin resistance and the body's ability to recognize and use insulin appropriately. Here is what happens when sugar cannot penetrate the cell because fat is in the way:

How Insulin Brings Sugar to the Cell

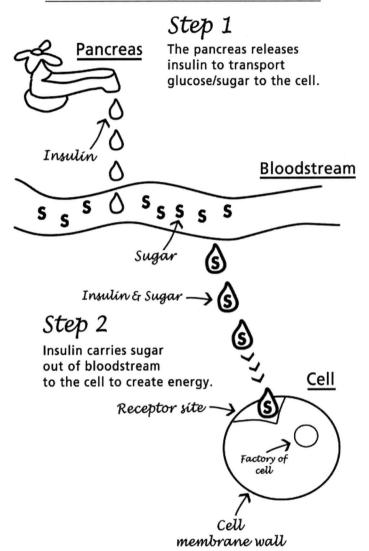

Step 1

Pancreas

The pancreas releases insulin to transport glucose/sugar to the cell.

Insulin

Bloodstream

Sugar

Insulin & Sugar →

Step 2

Insulin carries sugar out of bloodstream to the cell to create energy.

Cell

Receptor site →

Factory of cell

Cell membrane wall

How Fat Causes Adult-Onset Diabetes

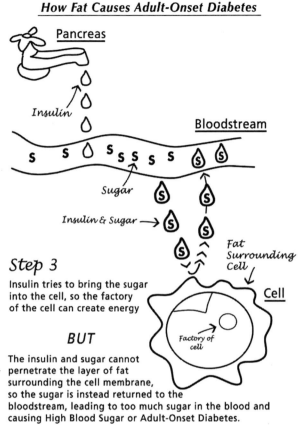

Pancreas

Insulin

Bloodstream

S   S   S S S S   S   S   S

Sugar

Insulin & Sugar →

Fat
Surrounding
Cell

Cell

Step 3

Insulin tries to bring the sugar
into the cell, so the factory
of the cell can create energy

*Factory of
cell*

BUT

The insulin and sugar cannot
pernetrate the layer of fat
surrounding the cell membrane,
so the sugar is instead returned to the
bloodstream, leading to too much sugar in the blood and
causing High Blood Sugar or Adult-Onset Diabetes.

So lose weight (body fat) to help prevent Adult-Onset Diabetes!

The good news is that people at risk for type 2 diabetes can prevent or delay developing diabetes by losing a little weight. The International Diabetes Foundation states that "there is substantial evidence that lifestyle changes *(achieving a healthy body weight and moderate physical activity)* can help prevent the development of type 2 diabetes and should be the initial intervention for all people at risk".[8] Hear that? A healthy lifestyle of exercise and eating right may actually help you avoid this disease!

Fat-Related Cancers

Prostate Cancer and Breast Cancer

The Harvard Nurses' Health Study found, after 12 years of following their participants, that greater consumption of red meat was strongly related to elevated risk of breast cancers.[9] Research that has tracked women who have emigrated from Japan to Hawaii or California has shown a six-fold increase in breast cancer when women moved to the United States.[10] In Japan, only one in 144 women has breast cancer. Further east, in the Hawaiian Islands, she becomes one in 15. If she continues her eastward movement to mainland U.S.A., then she becomes one in nine! The only change major difference is her diet. It was higher in fat in the U.S. than in her native country, Japan. She became influenced by our Western diet and some of our Western problems, such as breast cancer. Now is this definitive? No, but from an epidemiological *(population trends)* point of view, the type of fat and her body size began to change.

A recent article from the Journal of Women's Health noted "extensive data supports the hypothesis that a high-fat diet is conducive to the development of breast cancer in postmenopausal women."[11] The major commonality in studies about the effects of diet on breast cancer and prostate cancer is the frequent use of saturated and polyunsaturated fat in the diet. Populations that eat less saturated fat *(meat, high-fat dairy)* and less polyunsaturated fat *(vegetable oils, corn oil, etc.)* have lower prevalence of breast cancer in women and prostate cancer in men.

When looking at diet in conjunction with cancer of the prostate, saturated fat is the greatest evil. Randomized clinical trials have found that saturated fat may increase the risk of prostate cancer.[12] Cases of prostate cancer are more common in

Westernized countries, where saturated fat is more prevalent in the day to day diet. Incidences of prostate cancer also rose within Eastern countries as they started to become more "Westernized." Not surprisingly, there is also a correlation between the number of cases of prostate cancer and obesity.

"Red meats" such as beef, lamb and pork are thought to increase the risk of prostate cancer, as they contain a lot of fat *(up to as much as 30-40% in cuts from domesticated farm animals)*. Note: To clear up some confusion, although pork is not actually red in color, it is included in the "red meat" category by the United States Department of Agriculture *(USDA)* because its fat content is high, making it more similar to red meats than to white meats. Dairy products have also been linked to prostate cancer because of their high saturated fat content. Of course, dairy products are easily available in low-fat varieties as well.

Overall, it appears that high levels of saturated fat in the diet can greatly increase the risk of both prostate and breast cancer. Thus, making sure you have a healthy diet and keeping tabs on your intake of fat can help prevent or decrease your risk of these types of cancers *(sounds like it's worth it to me)*.

Colorectal Cancer

A high body mass index *(BMI, which is a height to weight ratio)*, high calorie intake, a lack of physical activity, and a larger waist size are all associated with colorectal cancer. A diet that is high in fruits, vegetables and grains, and low in saturated fats, is helpful in colorectal cancer prevention.

Vegetables and Fruits:

Red, yellow, orange and green-colored fruits and vegetables, such as peppers, oranges, strawberries and carrots, are particularly rich in a complex mixture of substances called antioxidants. Cruciferous vegetables *(cabbage, Brussels sprouts, broccoli, etc.)* have very high levels of these natural cancer-fighting chemicals. Brussels sprouts and broccoli are especially antioxidant-rich. There is increasing medical data that people who eat these foods, plus generous amounts of whole grains, have a lower risk of colon/colorectal cancer.

Meats and Saturated Fats:

Meat contains saturated fat, as do many processed products such as ice cream, pastries, rich sauces, etc. Always read the food labels to see how much saturated fat a food contains. These fats are broken down by the body's digestive juices and bile. Some of their byproducts are known to cause cancer in laboratory animals.

A study published in *Recent Results of Cancer Research* has shown that diets high in red and processed meat increase the risk of colorectal cancer.[13] A diet with reduced meat and saturated fat intake appears to contribute to colon health.

Fiber:

A high fiber diet acts like a broom, sweeping potentially toxic waste products through the intestines more quickly, thus reducing the time that the lining of the bowel walls are exposed to potential cancer-causing substances. Insoluble fiber *(the stringy stuff that holds plants together)* is found in the leaves, peels and skins of fruits and vegetables and in the exterior portion of whole grains *(such as wheat bran)*. Insoluble fiber cleans out your intestines like a brush. This is why it is crucial to choose whole-grain products *(such as whole wheat bread, brown rice, oatmeal, whole-grain pasta, whole-grain cereal, etc.)* instead of "white" or processed grain products *(such as white bread, white rice, white pasta, etc.)*. This is also why it is important to eat the skin of fruits and vegetables *(apples! potatoes! peaches! tomatoes! cucumber!)*

whenever possible. Do not cut that skin off! Of course, I'm not suggesting that you start chomping on banana or orange peels! Fiber also promotes colon health by discouraging the growth of harmful bacteria and encouraging the growth of beneficial bacteria.

In most Western countries, cancers of the bowel are the second most common type of cancer among men *(after lung cancer)*. However, in developing nations such as Africa, these bowel cancers are relatively rare. Dr. Dennis Burkitt, who won the Nobel Prize in the late 1960's for discovering Burkett's Lymphoma, attributed this discrepancy in part to the differences in diet between Western and African nations. Specifically, typical diets in Western nations consist of more refined/processed carbohydrates and contain less fiber than typical diets in African countries.[14]

A colorectal polyp is a growth on the inner wall of the colon or rectum. Polyps can cause bleeding and can, over time, develop into cancers. Polyps can be prevented by eating a diet that is low in fat and high in fruits, vegetables and fiber.[15]

Other Cancers

Obesity has also been linked to: cancer of the esophagus and gastric cardia, endometrial cancer, and renal cell cancer.

Arteriosclerosis
(Hardening of the Arteries)

You may have seen a picture of the yellow plaque that forms inside an artery. If you continue along the high-fat diet course, your arteries will continue to be filled with saturated fat. As you eat foods high in fat and gain weight, your body will produce more cholesterol. When the cholesterol combines with the saturated fat, artery blockage occurs.

Blockage of coronary arteries will decrease the blood flow to the heart. Decreased blood flow to the heart means lower levels of much-needed oxygen get to the heart. This lack of oxygen to the heart can cause chest pain *(angina)*, and a heart attack will follow if an artery is severely blocked. Similarly, a stroke results from inadequate blood flow to the brain, which can be caused by excessive accumulation of fatty plaque along the carotid artery walls.

Most diseases are significantly more manageable if caught early or better yet, if steps can be taken to prevent them once you find out you are at risk. In order to catch diseases early or find out if we are at risk, we must put aside our fears of medical offices and go to the doctor. When you go to the doctor to have a physical *(yes, you should do this regularly)*, your physician may recommend a series of blood tests.

Lipid Profile

One of these recommended blood tests may be a LIPID PROFILE. If it is not recommended, you may want to ask about it. This blood test will determine how much and what kinds of cholesterol and triglycerides your body is producing. If your total cholesterol production is more than 200, and your good cholesterol is not protecting you, the doctor will likely put you on a cholesterol-lowering medication as a precautionary measure to prevent the blockage.

The lipid profile will look like this:

	Desired Range
Total Cholesterol	100-199
HDL (good cholesterol)	40-59
LDL (bad cholesterol)	0-99
HDL/LDL Ratio	0.5-3.0
Triglycerides	0-149

Notes: HDL stands for "high density lipoprotein" and LDL stands for "low density lipoprotein." See chapter "Know Your Cholesterol"

Homocysteine Test

This is a fairly new test to detect if there is blockage in your arteries and, if so, to what extent. Homocysteine itself is an amino acid, which is suggested to damage the inner lining of the arteries and promote the fatty deposits in the blood vessels. As for now, this simple blood test is not routinely ordered with your Lipid Profile Test *(which includes total cholesterol, HDL, LDL, and triglycerides)*. You will need to ask your physician to order it. The range of results is 5-15, with desirable results being under 9. If your homocysteine level is too high, you may not be getting enough B vitamins to help your body use the homocysteine.

What to Do After You Get the Results

When you get the results of your profile back, you will have a picture of your situation. Many physicians will suggest you take a few months to change your diet around, in hopes of lowering your cholesterol. Others are tired of telling people to lose weight and eat right, so they will just hand you the medication, in order to decrease your chance for life-threatening heart problems. Of course, there are side effects of the various medications, which also vary among individuals *(as with any type of medication)*. The side effects are often worth dealing with, considering what the "side effects" are of not lowering your cholesterol. Unless your cholesterol is really elevated, you may want to do a little experiment of the effects of lifestyle on your individual cholesterol levels *(check with your doctor first)*.

Consider taking two months and really focusing on changing your eating habits and developing a regular exercise routine, as well as making an effort to manage your stress levels *(exercising is one way of doing this)*. Needless to say, smoking tobacco is also a major risk factor for high cholesterol. Schedule your next appointment in advance – so you do not forget or lose track of time – and see if your lipid profile changes for the better. If it does, you will have an idea of how much of your high cholesterol is due to behavioral issues that you have control over *(assuming you really did adopt a healthier lifestyle during those two months)*. However, if you get re-checked and your cholesterol is still too high, you will need to consider getting on the medication *(while also still continuing to adopt a healthier lifestyle)*. Some factors – like genetics – are not able to be changed behaviorally. Still, if you only lower your cholesterol production through taking the medication, while continuing to have unhealthy eating habits, your arteries will continue to be subjected to the heart attack and stroke-causing blockage. Thoroughly discuss with your doctor before deciding whether or not to take or to stop taking any medication.

Dr. Dean Ornish is probably one of the first research cardiologists to prove you can reverse blocked arteries through diet, without medication. He did a one-year and later a five-year study, published in the *Journal of the American Medical Association*, which showed that proper diet opened the blockage up to 30% and allowed a 300% greater volume of blood flow through these arteries.[16] His studies showed that by lowering your saturated fat intake and increasing your fiber intake, primarily from legumes and oat bran, you can reverse your blocked arteries with diet alone. Fantastic!

Exercise will also help you raise your HDL *(high density lipoprotein)* level, which is the good cholesterol. Omega-3 fatty acids from specific fish *(salmon, herring, sardines, anchovies and mackerel)* will help lower your triglycerides, which are a measure of fat and sugar produced by the liver. Tuna also contains adequate amounts of omega-3, although in somewhat lesser amounts than the other fish listed above. Meat, eggs and milk from grass-fed *(as opposed to grain-fed)* animals often have higher levels of omega-3, and many grocery stores now carry omega-3 rich eggs. Walnuts are also a good source of omega-3.

So the take home message, to help prevent you from ending up in the hospital, is: Lower your weight; back off the saturated fat; eat more legumes and whole grains for fiber; get rid of your sedentary lifestyle, and you will help unblock those arteries. Go for it! You CAN do it!

Hypoglycemia *(Low Blood Sugar)*

When your blood sugar level drops too low to provide enough energy for your body's activities, that's called hypoglycemia or low blood sugar.

Mild hypoglycemia is usually caused by skipping meals or waiting too long to eat. When your blood sugar drops, you may experience symptoms such as: light headedness, irritability, shakiness, headaches, perspiration, loss of energy, heightened emotionality, sleepiness, anxiety and loss of mental alertness. When this occurs, people scramble for food, any food. "I want food and I want it now!" said your body to your brain.

If you allow your blood sugar to drop too low, emotion overtakes reason, and you grab whatever is there, because you need to eat NOW. Following your quick gorge on the local cheeseburger, you may proceed to "beat yourself up" for being out of control and then determine that you're a failure. You just blew your "diet," so what the heck, you might as well keep blowing it. "Monday, we'll start again," said the dieter to her body.

But it does not have to be like that. Staying on a regular eating routine, eating breakfast, and eating more complex carbohydrates *(especially whole grain foods)* instead of simple carbohydrates *(foods and drinks with added sugar, but also food made with "white" or refined flour, etc.)* will help your blood sugar remain steady for longer. Think of what happens after drinking a soda: you get that "sugar high" which may briefly give you some increased energy. That, by the way, is only useful if you are actually able to concentrate on your sugar high. But soon after, your blood sugar quickly drops, and that sugar high morphs into a "sugar low," making you feel less productive and even worse than before. Moral of the story: It is not worth it! Do not let yourself get to that point where you grab anything and eat before you have time to think.

Everyone experiences symptoms of hypoglycemia at some point. But hypoglycemia can also be a pathologic condition that may require special medical attention and proper diet. If you experience any of these symptoms mentioned above on a regular basis, then you should request a five-hour glucose tolerance test. This will usually show if you have functional *(reactive)* hypoglycemia. Have your doctor ask the lab technician who administers the test to observe and discuss your physical symptoms with you during the test. Normal fasting blood sugar levels range from 70 to 110 mg/dl. So lower than 70 usually indicates hypoglycemia.

The cause and treatment of functional *(reactive)* hypoglycemia are still open to debate, but there are behaviors you can do to help relieve the symptoms of both more and less serious types of hypoglycemia. The behaviors include eating small meals or snacks every three hours, exercising regularly, eating well-balanced meals that include high fiber foods, and avoiding sugary foods or drinks.

Premenstrual Syndrome - Pms
(or "Pretty Mean Streak," as a foolish husband once said)

Premenstrual Syndrome is the name of a group of symptoms that start 7 to 14 days before a women's period *(menstruation)*. The symptoms usually stop shortly after one's period begins. Physical and emotional symptoms are many and variable and could include anxiety, irritability, depression, bloating, painful cramping, acne, nausea, headache, backache, gastrointestinal problems, and a marked increase of carbohydrate cravings.

A nurse and friend of mine, alleges "PMS is what men have all the time!" In any case, there are so many bad jokes and so much misleading information about PMS that many do not know what to believe. Some women say they never experience it, while numerous others say, "Honey, you just look at me wrong, and I'll bite your 'friggin' head off." OK, let's talk about this. And yes, you men need to continue reading too.

Exactly what causes PMS is unknown, but several risk factors may contribute to the condition. Hormonal fluctuations, chemical changes in the brain, and diet are contributors to this often joked about condition. Many a woman and man have often wondered why appetites seem out of control and willpower goes out the window during PMS. We must understand that factors such as brain chemicals and fluctuations in hormone production exert powerful influences over behavior and physical cravings.

The week prior to a woman's menstrual cycle, the pancreas produces greater amounts of insulin than any other time during the month. Insulin's job is to transport glucose *(sugar)*, whether from starches or simple sugars, out of the bloodstream and into the cells for the production of energy. Thus, with greater amounts of insulin in the blood, larger amounts of sugar are transported out of the blood and into the cells, resulting in a severe drop of the blood sugar. As discussed earlier, in relation to hypoglycemia, there are a plethora of not-so-fun symptoms that may occur in response to low blood sugar. As a result of the drop, the individual may also experience cravings for more sugar.

A good way to help lessen the severity of both hypoglycemic and PMS symptoms, particularly while trying to stay on a healthy diet regimen, is to become quite routine with your meal times. This will prevent the ol' drop of the blood sugar. Plan and eat five small meals daily, all based on starch, whole grains or complex carbohydrates *(slow-acting carbohydrates)*. Note the word "small" in the recommended "five small meals daily." Obviously, if you are going from eating three to five meals daily, you will have to develop a slightly new perspective on what a "typical" meal size is.

For example, the five "meals" could be: breakfast, mid-morning snack, lunch, afternoon snack, supper, and possibly a sixth small evening snack. The snacks could be: cereal/granola bars, toast with jam and/or a small amount of peanut butter, whole-grain crackers *(WASA crackers, Trisquits, Wheat-thins)* or a little *(1/2 cup)* cereal with low-fat yogurt or low-fat milk.

Suggestions for those who suffer from PMS include the following:

- Eat complex carbohydrates *(such as whole-grain breads, pastas and cereals)*, fiber and protein.
- Cut back on sugar and fat.
- Avoid salt for the last few days before your period to reduce bloating and fluid retention, and drink plenty of water.
- Try eating up to six small meals a day instead of three larger ones.
- Cut out or down on alcohol, to decrease feelings of depression

- Exercise 30 minutes, 4-6 times a week. It will actually help alleviate cramping.
- Get plenty of sleep, about 8 hours a night. Make more effort than usual to get to bed on time, just for this week.
- Keep a regular schedule of meals, bedtime and exercise.
- If you tend to become highly emotional during this time, you may want to refrain from making any major decisions until after the symptoms have subsided.

- Take Vitamin B6. Today there are numerous OB/GYN physicians who recommend taking vitamin B6 *(200 mg daily)* 7-10 days prior to the menstrual cycle. The reason is that vitamin B6, or pyrodoxine, converts to serotonin, a neurotransmitter that causes the release of endorphins *(the brain's opiates)*, which make us feel relaxed and calm. Taking vitamin B6 seems to help the mood swings to level out.

Sleep Apnea

Many of my overweight and obese clients have sleep apnea. Among patients with obstructive sleep apnea, at least 60-70% are obese. In fact, obesity – particularly upper-body obesity – is the most significant risk factor for obstructive sleep apnea. There is actually a 12 to 30-fold increase of this disorder among people with morbid obesity as compared to the general population.[17] Obstructive sleep apnea *(OSA)* is a disorder in which extra fatty tissue around the upper airway causes a person to stop breathing during the night, perhaps even hundreds of times, usually for 10 seconds or longer.

In many cases, the person may be unaware of it, but his/her bed partner is not. Loud snoring and gasps for breath may alert and scare the bed partner, while disrupting the partner's sleep. Symptoms the person with sleep apnea may experience include excessive daytime sleepiness, morning headaches and irritability.

When you stop breathing, your brain does not get enough oxygen. As a result of this lack of oxygen and lack of sleep, drastic problems can arise. Some of these problems may include: heart problems, stroke, high blood pressure, depression, memory loss and an increased risk of auto accidents. Patients may need to consult a sleep specialist if a sleep history and physical exam does not diagnose suspected sleep apnea.

Many diagnosed with sleep apnea end up having to sleep while wearing a mask that is connected to a CPAP *(continuous positive airway pressure)* machine which sits next to their bed. This machine keeps the airway open and helps the person breathe. HOWEVER, weight loss may alleviate the need for a CPAP machine. Overweight individuals who lose even 10% of their weight may reduce sleep apnea, while dramatically improving their quality of life, sleep and health *(and probably that of their partner's as well)*.

Hypertension

High blood pressure, or hypertension, is simply the condition that occurs when the pressure of the blood in your arteries is too high. Hypertension has been called "the silent killer" because of two reasons: (1) the only way you can know if you have it is to get your blood pressure checked *(which is now one of the most common procedures done in health care facilities)* and (2) high blood pressure greatly increases your risk for stroke, heart attack, heart failure, and kidney failure. High blood pressure is very common in our society, but is especially common among people who are overweight or obese. The risk of developing high blood pressure is 5 to 6 times greater in obese adult Americans ages 20 to 45, in comparison to non-obese individuals of the same age. Furthermore, over 75% of reported hypertension cases are attributed directly to obesity.[17]

The epidemic of obesity in the United States contributes to the prevalence of hypertension among children, adolescents and adults of all racial/ethnic groups and of both genders. Although widely common among all groups, hypertension occurs with even higher prevalence among minority populations, especially among African Americans, who tend to experience an earlier onset and a more severe course of hypertension.[18]

When you have your blood pressure tested, you can do certain things to increase the accuracy of the test, including avoiding food, alcohol, caffeine, and tobacco in the 30 to 60 minutes prior to the test. It is also a good idea to be seated for 5 minutes, breathing deeply and trying to relax, before being tested. This prevents artificially inflated readings due to anxiety from being at the doctor's office or due to having it taken immediately after walking around. To be sure your results are reliable, you should also have your blood pressure taken on more than one occasion.

Blood pressure is represented by two numbers, one on the top and one on the bottom. A pressure of 120/80 is usually read as "120 over 80." The number on top is the systolic pressure, which means the pressure in your arteries when your heart beats, and the number on the bottom is the diastolic pressure, which means the pressure in your arteries when your heart is resting between beats. Optimal blood pressure is usually considered to be 120/80, although some people may have lower blood pressure. Generally, hypertension is considered to be present when someone's systolic pressure is consistently above 140 or when someone's diastolic pressure is consistently above 90, or both. Of course, guidelines for diagnosis may vary from person to person and from doctor to doctor. Individuals with pre-existing conditions, such as diabetes, may be cautioned at even lower numbers.

Thankfully, hypertension is treatable. Individuals with blood pressure only slightly higher than normal may be able to treat it through lifestyle changes alone. These lifestyle changes include: eating healthy, exercising, decreasing salt intake, not drinking more than two alcoholic drinks per day, increasing calcium and potassium in your diet, and of course, not smoking. Individuals with markedly high blood pressure, or whose high blood pressure does not respond enough to lifestyle changes, can take medications that effectively lower the blood pressure. Still, it is widely-recognized that the number one thing that can be done to prevent and to alleviate high blood pressure is adopting a healthier lifestyle *(which includes maintaining a healthy weight).*

Osteoarthritis

Osteoarthritis is the most common type of arthritis. It causes the cartilage in a joint to become stiff and lose elasticity. Over time, the cartilage breaks down, forcing ligaments to stretch and bones to rub against each other. The result is pain and loss of joint movement.

There have been many studies on the association between obesity and osteoarthritis. There is a strong correlation between this type of arthritis and affected weight-bearing joints, like your hips, back and knees. The extra weight placed on these joints, particularly the knees and hips, results in rapid wear and tear and pain caused by inflammation.

Weight loss has been found to be a practical and favorable treatment in the rehabilitation of patients with knee osteoarthritis. Weight loss reduces physical pressure on the joints and bones. According to the American Obesity Association, modest weight loss of 10 to 15 pounds is likely to relieve symptoms and delay disease progression of knee osteoarthritis.[17] Maintaining a recommended weight helps prevent osteoarthritis and reduces stress on your weight-bearing joints. Gentle exercise, such as swimming or walking on flat surfaces, helps improve joint movement and strengthen the muscles surrounding these joints. Obesity has also been found to be related to the development of rheumatoid arthritis, in both men and women.

Osteoporosis

Osteoporosis, or "porous bones," is the weakening of bones caused by an imbalance between bone building and bone destruction. Calcium is a mineral that the body needs for numerous functions, including building and maintaining bones and teeth. So you've heard about the little old lady who crossed the street, fell and broke her hip? Her diagnosis: osteoporosis. Her hip had lost bone density. Then she fell. The suspected cause: Lack of calcium weakened her bones. In reality, she may or may not have been getting enough calcium throughout her life. Most likely, the cause was actually...drum roll please...too much protein.

As previously stated, in America, we typically eat too much protein. Protein competes with calcium for absorption, and when protein competes with calcium for absorption, protein wins. Since the 1920's, researchers have known that diets that are high in protein, especially animal protein, can cause excessive amounts of calcium to be lost through the urine (*i.e. you eliminate it instead of absorbing it).*[19] In nations – including our own – with high rates of osteoporosis, protein intake is generally also high, usually more than twice the recommended daily allowance. Countries whose citizens tend to have diets lower in protein have fewer incidences of hip fractures and of osteoporosis.[20] But wait, there's more. Not only does a diet high in protein cause you to lose more calcium, it also puts you at an increased risk for developing kidney stones! This is no recent discovery; nearly thirty years ago, British researchers found that adding 34 grams of additional protein to a normal diet resulted in increasing the risk of urinary tract stones by as much as 250 percent![21]

Read more about calcium in the chapter titled "Vitamins, Minerals, and Water."

Other Health Effects

According to the American Obesity Association, other diseases and health conditions that overweight/obesity have been linked to include:[17]

- Birth defects
- Carpal Tunnel Syndrome
- Chronic Venous Insufficiency *(inadequate blood flow through the veins)*
- Daytime sleepiness
- Deep Vein Thrombosis *(blood clots in your leg)*
- End Stage Renal Disease
- Gallbladder Disease
- Gout
- Heat Disorders
- Impaired Immune Response
- Impaired Respiratory Function
- Infections following wounds
- Infertility
- Liver Disease
- Low Back Pain
- Obstetric and Gynecologic Complications
- Pain *(general)*
- Pancreatitis
- Stroke
- Surgical Complications
- Urinary Stress Incontinence

The Partnership Program

Often it helps when two people in the same household, or two friends or two co-workers, go on the program together. They motivate each other, help each other, and even badger each other to "do the right thing." I have seen this work well with couples, a parent and child, or even a group of friends who walk together and meet weekly for reinforcement. This mutual support allows them to share feelings, thoughts, and frustrations with someone who really understands what they are going through. Everyone wants to have someone to moan and groan with every once in while!

Partnership with Spouse or Significant Other

I had a very nice Hispanic couple come into my office for nutritional counseling. The husband, a former high school track athlete, had grown from 165 pounds to 210 pounds, while his diminutive wife had blossomed from 118 pounds to 168 pounds over their 20 years of marriage. They both felt ready to make some healthy changes in their lives, which is, in itself, an important first step. Without each others' support, it would have been quite difficult, if not impossible. They decided to hold each other accountable by making sure they ate supper together, usually Monday through Friday. In case they didn't feel like cooking, they kept the refrigerator stocked with low-fat, tasty frozen entrees and made a large salad to go along with it. As long as they ate the same meal at dinner, one didn't feel as if the other was getting something better or more desirable. On most nights before supper, they power-walked through the neighborhood together. They agreed to meet at home at a set time, despite their busy schedules, to walk and have a meal. This became their routine.

Making such an agreement and sticking to it is important. Let's say you make an effort to get home from work by your specific, agreed upon time, and 20 minutes later your partner still hasn't shown up. You get frustrated and begin to lose the motivation you had a hard time mustering up in the first place. The agreement has been ruined and many undesirable outcomes occur: you didn't walk while waiting for him/her, or maybe you snacked a lot while you were waiting because you knew you would be eating dinner later, or you got frustrated and started feeling negatively toward that person. Whatever the outcome, it usually isn't good. Of course, everyone runs late or has things come up occasionally, but it is extremely important to maintain the routine and uphold the agreement, in order for you both to keep your motivation and for the partnership to work.

So agree to meet, do it, walk, eat right and be healthy! Rely on each other, and know that when you uphold that agreement, you are "being there" for both your partner and yourself.

It worked for the couple above. A year and a half after completing my program, the wife is maintaining her weight at 128 pounds, while the husband is staying between 160 to 165 pounds. They feel better about themselves, more confident about their health, and proud that they have accomplished something together.

Partnership Between Parent and Child

Many parents first become motivated to make healthier decisions because they are concerned about their children's weight and how being overweight might affect them. There is no way children can accomplish weight loss on their own. In the past, I have seen many parents come into my office with their 10 year-old or 14 year-old overweight child. Usually, the parents are also overweight, yet some parents never admit that they too are overweight and may be contributing to the child's physical condition. In order for the child to lose weight, the parents must start the program too, but they are not always willing. We cannot expect kids to take full responsibility for their weight and health. Without the support of the people who buy the food, make the dinners and set the rules, children will most likely fail at losing weight. Without parents acting as positive influences and modeling how to make healthy choices, kids who gain plenty of nutrition knowledge still fail at losing weight. It's really not fair.

Often, I ask the child to help the parent(s). I purposely do this in the beginning to give the child a sense of responsibility. This can work to facilitate a "give-and-take" between parent(s) and child. Difficulty usually arises when the child is overbooked with after-school activities and has no time to exercise, or if the parents will not adjust their work demands to be there for the child's exercise needs. Most often, the most difficult part of the weight loss process for the child is exercising. Brisk walking is the best fat burner. However, the child may not see the benefit, think it's "un-cool" and give the parent a difficult time. Deals can be made to entice the child, if necessary. This is a common tactic and can work well if implemented properly and if the parent does not falter on the agreement.

For example, a deal could be a monetary incentive: "Walk with me five days a week, and I'll pay you a dollar/two dollars for each walk. If you walk all five days, I'll give you a bonus dollar." Alternatively, you could promise the child a trip to the movies or shopping over the weekend if he/she walks all five days. Another alternative is an hour or two of television watching for the night if the child walks and none if he/she doesn't. In this case, at least if the child does not walk, it is not because of watching TV. Remember, if you make a deal, you must keep it. The first time you break the deal and do not follow through, your child will lose motivation and the "deal-making" strategy will no longer be effective. PS – don't make food the reward!

The message here: Set aside the time and make the effort to partner with your kid. Your child is one of the best motivators for you to become healthier. You want to be around to see them graduate high school, college, get married and have children, don't you? You making healthier decisions is the number one thing you can do to make it easier for your child to be healthier. The whole family will reap the benefits.

Walking Partners

Obviously, this is a good idea. But beware; an unreliable partner who becomes a "no show" can become your excuse for not walking yourself. So choose wisely.

One "deal" or agreement I recommend is a contract, even in writing, with your walking partner. We are talking money here! For example: You both agree to meet at a certain place and time, for a specific five days, say Monday through Friday at 6 p.m. at the high school track. Whoever doesn't show up that day pays the other $5. To begin with, make the contract for two weeks.

Another "deal" that works for couples or roommates is the "Clean Bathroom Deal." This deal is that you must show up five days in a row and the first to miss cleans the bathroom! Now there's a good source of motivation! Figure out what kind of deal will work best for you and your partner.

The Vegetarian in the Crowd

There are so many questions and misinformation about this subject. "Will becoming a vegetarian help me lose weight?" "Will I get enough protein and how?" "Is it healthier?" "As a vegetarian, I can't eat out, there's nothing on the menu!" "How do I balance my foods?" "I've heard it is difficult..."

Is vegetarianism a lifestyle or just a healthier way of eating? In 1968, vegetarianism was hip and the country's awareness on all levels was changing. A major war was on, change was everywhere, and the realization of our resources and our existence being finite sparked a different kind of awareness. The food bible of the '60s, *Diet for a Small Planet*, by Frances Moore Lappe, hit the bookstores. This became the guide on how to become ecologically aware of the inefficient way we were eating.

What do I mean by "the inefficient way we were eating"? Some interesting facts that you have probably never thought about are: In the production of chicken for food, it takes 6 pounds of corn to grow 1 pound of chicken. In the production of cattle for food, it takes 30 pounds of corn to grow 1 pound of beef! Meat began to be viewed, by some, as not only a very expensive protein source but also as a less efficient way to use our resources and an industry that resulted in the overuse of fertilizers and pesticides.

Some people became vocal about being against killing animals for food. People became more aware that they could get the protein needed for growth, digestion and maintenance of body tissues and cells from plant sources and that meat was not completely necessary for survival and good health.

Vegetarianism in the '60s bore a close resemblance to a true low-fat diet. In fact, cut out the meat and lessen the dairy products and there goes most of the saturated fats we eat. There was no such existence of tons of "fat-free" products lining the grocery store aisles, but they did have "animal-free" and therefore, a low-fat diet. Some years later, Tufts University's Dr. Johanna Dwyer created an epidemiological study using a mostly vegetarian religious community of the Seventh Day Adventists.

Dr. Dwyer studied the frequency and occurrence of heart disease and various forms of cancer and obesity in both this vegetarian community and in a sample of the general population. Her findings revealed that the vegetarian Seventh Day Adventists were significantly healthier than the rest of our population. Their incidence of heart disease occurred 10 years later in life than the national average. The incidence of stomach cancer, colorectal cancer, breast cancer, and prostate cancer was much lower. There were fewer obese people as well.

They also lived longer than their carnivorous *(meat-eating)* counterparts. Why? They were not eating as much fat or protein as the rest of America and as a result, had fewer health problems. Evidence today is mounting against fat. Cut back on fat, and you improve your chances of not having these diet-related diseases.

Balanced/Complimentary Proteins

The bean said to the rice, "Oh rice, I like your amino acids a lot," and the rice replied, "Oh, Mr. Bean, you always compliment me!" Or as in the movie *Jerry Maguire*, "You complete me." In fact, these cheesy jokes are actually quite accurate.

As discussed in the beginning of this book, most people in the world eat starches: rice, noodles, beans, peas, lentils, bread, cereal, corn, and barley, to name a few. What many Americans do not know is that specific amino acids *(proteins)* are present in every starch. Grains *(rice, noodles, bread)* have different kinds of protein than legumes *(beans and peas)* have and in lesser amounts. But interestingly enough, if you put the grains and legumes together, they give you a complete protein. There is a total of 22 different kinds of amino acids that the body needs. Fourteen are made by the body, so eight need to come from the diet. Thus, these eight are called the "essential amino acids."

All animal protein *(meat, dairy, egg, poultry and fish)* have the eight essential amino acids and thus, are called "complete proteins." Neither grains nor legumes are complete by themselves. However, if you eat them both *(either in the same meal or at least during the same day)*, they become complete proteins! Yes, the same quality protein as in a sirloin steak, but with much less fat and more fiber!

These are examples of how you can combine different kinds of legumes and grains in the same meal: beans and rice, lima beans and cornbread, pasta and beans *(an Italian dish, called "Pasta Fagioli")* or hummus and bread. When mentioning beans, we're talking: black beans, red beans, pinto beans, lima beans, kidney beans, soy beans, and navy beans, but not green *(or string)* beans. Black-eyed peas are also included in this category, although green *(English)* peas are not. Legumes and grains should be consumed in a one-to-one ratio, such as one cup of beans to one cup of rice, or 1/2 cup of pasta to 1/2 cup of beans. Balancing proteins, as stated in *Diet for a Small Planet*, is not difficult.

An example of a well-balanced, meatless meal could be black beans with rice and a salad *(or another green vegetable)*. For more flavor, add a little salsa, low-fat cheese or low-fat sour cream, hot sauce, or diced onions, green peppers and tomatoes. Especially if you are from the South, you may have heard of a dish called "Hoppin' John," the traditional New Year's Day meal of black-eyed peas and rice that is supposed to bring good luck for the New Year! Adding salsa or Pickapeppa sauce is a low-fat alternative to ham hocks for flavoring, and may contribute even more good luck for the coming year...at least as far as your health is concerned. An example with a Mexican influence is a bean burrito with low-fat refried beans on a corn or wheat tortilla. Again, good toppings are salsa, low-fat cheese or low-fat sour cream, hot sauce, diced onions and tomatoes and/or chopped lettuce. The brand "Mission" makes whole-grain flour tortillas. Try them next time you are making a quick and easy Mexican dinner.

Tip to Remember: When you combine a grain *(rice, pasta, corn and bread)* with a legume *(beans, peas and lentils)* in a 1:1 ratio, you have a complete protein, the same quality protein as beef but with much less fat.

Types of Vegetarians

Lacto-Ovo or Lacto Vegetarian

A lacto-ovo vegetarian is a person who does not eat meat but does eat dairy *("lacto")* products, such as cheese, yogurt, milk and eggs *("ovo")*. The lacto vegetarian eats dairy but does not eat eggs.

Vegan

People who are vegan do not eat any animal products at all, no eggs or dairy and nothing made with any amount of eggs or dairy. For most people, this type of lifestyle is pretty radical. But ironically, this way of eating eliminates all animal fats, including all the saturated *(bad for your arteries)* fats. Basically, this diet consists of grains, legumes *(beans)*, fruits and vegetables. Other vegan sources of protein besides grains and legumes include nuts *(any kind, includes peanut butter)* and soy products *(such as tofu, soy milk, soy-based veggie burgers)*. One can use different kinds of sauces *(A-1, soy, salsa)* to make dishes with a variety of flavors.

Pescetarian *(or Pesco-Vegetarian)*

Whether or not this should actually be considered a type of vegetarianism is debated, but a pesco-vegetarian eats fish and non-mammalian seafood, but not meat *(no mammals or birds)*. Dairy and eggs may be part of a pesco-vegetarian diet as well. Fish is a low-fat and good source of protein, with many nutritional benefits.

My Opinion

From a strictly nutritional point of view, between choosing to be vegan or lacto vegetarian, I think lacto vegetarian, with low-fat dairy products, is the ticket. Drink skim or 1% milk *(or soymilk)* instead of whole, and choose low-fat cheeses and yogurts. This way, you are sure to get the calcium that you need. If you balance proteins correctly, growth and tissue repair is not a problem. The lacto vegetarian diet is healthy for children as well as adults, as long as attention is paid to making sure that meals are balanced and include a protein source. For adults and children, go with low-fat or even non-fat dairy products, but pediatricians still recommend 2% or whole-milk products for infants up to 2 years old.

Thinking About Making the Change or Want More Information?

Yes, being vegetarian is a major lifestyle commitment and one that requires you to educate yourself a bit and become open to a variety of foods. The teenager who suddenly announces that she has become vegetarian, but does not like vegetables, will not try new foods, and eats mainly meatless junk foods is NOT a good example of what it is to be vegetarian...in fact, she may be just joining a fad or on her way to an eating disorder. But anyone *(including teenagers)* who is serious about becoming vegetarian can do so, get enough protein, and be healthy...the key is to educate oneself on how to get a balanced diet. For more information, go to the bookstore and pick up a book on vegetarianism and a vegetarian cook book. You can also order "Vegetarian Starter Kits" that provide you with all the needed information at websites such as *VegetarianStarterKit.com* or *VegSource.com*.

Although only a small percentage of the American population is vegetarian and becoming totally vegetarian might be something you would never in a million years consider doing, we can ALL benefit from incorporating vegetarian meals into our diets and adopting the perspective that not every meal needs to contain *(or be centered around)* meat. Concentrating on having one or two vegetarian meals per week is likely to lessen your fat intake and prompt you to eat a greater variety of foods that are higher in vitamins and fiber *(vegetables, legumes, etc.)*. Even if a meatless meal sounds ludicrous to you right now, it will soon become "not so big a deal" and will help you focus more on the "other food groups."

Gastric Bypass Surgery

Today, many people who have 100 pounds or more to lose are requesting a surgery that creates a smaller stomach, limiting the amount one can consume. This radical surgery is certainly an alternative for people who are morbidly obese *(yes, this is a technical term)*. But, it has its drawbacks and is not as straightforward of a solution as it may seem. I have counseled numerous people who have opted for this surgery and thus, I well-understand and have compassion for those who seek it.

Gastric bypass and gastroplasty both reroute the digestive system. Gastroplasty also restricts the amount of food that can be eaten by making the stomach smaller. They are both considered non-reversible and require a 5 to 6 inch incision and a hospital stay of three to four days.

The newer lap band technique places a silicone band around the upper part of the stomach. The "down-sized" smaller upper stomach pouch limits the amount of food that can be consumed at one time. The stomach outlet is also narrowed, which increases the amount of time it takes for the stomach to empty.

Losing weight and keeping it off are some of the most difficult things people can do. Discipline, will-power, desire and focus are of utmost importance, particularly for those who are 100 or more pounds overweight. The task is daunting. Yet, I have had clients come in at 435 pounds and lose 235 pounds over a three-year period on my program *(without the surgery)* and keep it off for years after. I know it can be done.

That being said, gastric surgery can "do it for you" if you

cannot do it on your own, but you will still have to make healthy lifestyle changes after the surgery *(maybe more than you think)* in order to maintain its effectiveness and prevent other associated health problems.

The Pluses and Minuses

All three surgeries mentioned come with the need to be monitored after surgery and a necessary lifestyle change in diet and exercise. You may also need to take supplemental vitamins and minerals. And of course, they all come with possible surgical risks and potential serious complications, from malabsorption to blood clots, to leaking at surgical sites, to slippage of the lap band, to infection and possibly even death.

These surgeries are also expensive. If all goes well - no infections, no further complications – $25,000 is the most recent estimate I have heard for the gastric bypass. With complications, it can double. Who pays? Most people cannot afford this, so they badger their HMO or insurance company, which is also generally reluctant to spend the money. Or, they may seek help from a governmental agency such as Vocational Rehabilitation. Basically, the public, one way or the other, often pays. That's you and me.

The danger of postoperative complications and risks are always looming. I would say that if you are between 300 and 350 pounds, you have a better chance of surviving the surgery than if you are heavier. If you are over 350 pounds, your chances diminish considerably. Of course, operative risks always vary from person to person, and you must speak with a medical specialist to determine what yours are.

A Personal Anecdote from My Practice

Here is a story from the "front lines": I counseled a married couple who were in their late 40s and early 50s. Both wanted the surgery. The wife weighed 350 pounds, and the husband weighed 487 pounds. The wife had her operation before I met them, but the husband was told that he must lose 100 pounds before the HMO would pay for his surgery. These two very nice people showed up at my door after the wife's surgery because she was having severe abdominal discomfort and bowel distress daily. She was experiencing projectile vomiting and diarrhea constantly. She had been back to the surgeon's office and dietitian numerous times for help, but to no avail. *(Oh, and yes, by the way, she was in fact losing weight.)* The husband said he was desperate to lose weight and still wanted to have the surgery, despite watching his wife's suffering.

For the wife, I recommended a high-fiber, high-starch, frequent-feeding program that calls for very small portions. In less than a week, her gastro-intestinal problems had ceased. The husband, in turn, had started weight loss counseling with me and had begun to lose weight. His knees were in terrible shape, as you can imagine at 487 pounds. I tried to get him to go into a pool and "water walk." *(Remember what water walking is? If not, you can go to the chapter on walking to review.)* He was losing weight gradually, about 8 pounds per month. He would not dare get into a pool to water walk. He walked some with his wife, but his knees hurt severely. His wife was losing a lot of weight after the surgery and with the improvements in her diet.

The wife's former dietitian had recommended that, after the surgery, she eat small amounts of animal protein, which had contributed to the vomiting, etc. I suggested she eat no animal protein for a month and instead, consume grains and beans in small amounts, as well as more fruits and vegetables. This worked and totally changed her gastrointestinal functioning for the better.

Meanwhile, the husband's frustration mounted as he saw his wife's weight loss success and improved health. He desperately pushed for the operation. He had so far lost 30 pounds in about four months. His wife had lost about 60 pounds. Finally, the government agency relented and paid for the operation. He had the surgery on a Monday morning. By Thursday, he was complaining of severe pain in his abdominal area. The surgeon went back in and discovered an infection but could not find the source. By Friday evening, five days post-op, he was dead. He was a nice man, a loving husband and father, and dead at 50. What a shame. This influenced me even more to encourage others to try to lose weight without surgery.

His wife, in her grief, continued to lose down to 212 pounds from 350 in the year I had known her. Yet, her life had radically changed. At the last session we had, although saddened by her loss, she was still walking regularly and eating healthy.

The family is now suing the surgeon. Should the surgeon have done it, knowing the risks involved for this patient *(because of his size, among other things)*, or is it solely in the patient's hands for insisting that it be done? Either way, the damage has already been done.

It Can Be Frustrating

I well remember a newspaper article about a young 33 year-old mother who weighed 306 pounds. She was bound and determined to have gastric surgery. Her HMO, which has a protocol on who receives the operation, had sent her to me to first try nutrition and lifestyle counseling before they would authorize the surgery. She came to me only twice because she had already made up her mind that all she wanted was the operation. It was frustrating for both of us, because she certainly had no interest in what I had to tell her. My information, of course, was dealing with changing her habits, exercising, changing behavior and living a healthier lifestyle.

After the first two sessions, I never saw her again or heard about her until one day I read a newspaper article on how she had had the surgery and lost 120 pounds. It also explained what she was doing to lose more and keep it off. It sounded astonishingly familiar...She was now walking five times a week, eating a low-calorie, high-fiber, high-complex carbohydrate diet. My thoughts, after reading this were, "Duh!" It was what I asked her to do in the first place! Sure, it certainly would have taken longer to lose the weight through lifestyle changes alone, but she would have certainly avoided some pain, risk, and misery. According to the article, she had almost died twice of infection and complications from the surgery. Her family was traumatized. The photo accompanying the article showed her two young daughters walking with her. How close they came to losing their mother seems sad, scary, and unnecessary.

"Spit Out Chicken"

Another client who had the gastric surgery and who was also ill-advised on what she should eat post-surgery devised a unique method of eating. She had weighed in at around 350 pounds. After the surgery, she was experiencing diarrhea and vomiting. She went on my starch-based, higher-fiber, low-animal protein diet, and she was doing great. She was losing weight with no gastric side effects. She told me that once in a while she tried chicken and continued to get the same violent side effects. She also was very good about writing a daily food record.

I asked her what she really liked about eating chicken or meat. She, of course, replied, "The taste, dummy." *(OK, so she didn't really* say *"dummy."*) In any case, we devised a radical but appropriate-for-the-situation idea of putting a piece of chicken in her mouth, chewing it, enjoying the flavor, and then spitting it out. Now, please understand I am not a fan of bulimia and am not one to typically encourage this type of behavior, just a practical person who can revert to odd creativity when in dire straights.

Weeks later, she came into my office with her daily written record. As I read it I noticed one entry that read "Spit out chicken." At first, I did not realize what this was, and then it hit me. She had done it. She would cook her favorite chicken dish, sit down at the table and enjoy the taste, then spit it out! I didn't ask her if she was dining alone... I assumed so.

A few months later, at Easter, she entered this in her daily written record: "Spit out ham, sweet potatoes, green beans" (*she ate and could digest the sweet potatoes and green beans, just not the meat*). I understood the situation. It worked for her and her unique situation. This is not something I would generally recommend, but hey, it worked despite the oddity. She eventually could eat, swallow and digest small amounts of animal protein without getting sick.

My Conclusion

Gastric surgery is a very complicated decision for those eligible for it, but I truly believe it is possible to lose a significant amount of weight, even if one is morbidly obese, through lifestyle change alone. At least give it a real honest-to-goodness shot (*with real commitment*) before resorting to the surgical table.

How to Eat Out Without Pigging Out

What happens when you are on a weight loss program and a friend suggests going out to eat? You would love to go, but you fear losing control of your eating habits and eating too much. After all, the portions at restaurants in this country tend to be humongous! Can you actually go out, have fun, choose a healthy option and maintain control? Yes, you can!

Here is a scenario: You and your spouse are dining at a restaurant. He is 6'1" tall and weighs 220 pounds. You are 5'4" tall and weigh 155 pounds. You both decide to order the same entree. Why? Since your sizes are so different, should you have the same amount of food on your plates? Shouldn't each person get a portion of food corresponding to body size? The chefs, of course, do not approach it this way.

But you have options. You need to learn to control your eating environment.

You DO Have Options

Here are a few options for handling the large entrées restaurants tend to serve:

1. Split an Entrée
You and your dinner companion agree to split an order. You

tell the server: "We would like the blackened fish, baked potato and vegetable, and we would like you to put the entree on two separate plates, please. We would appreciate an extra salad and the house dressing on the side. Do you have cottage cheese, salsa, or an A-1 type sauce for the baked potato? That's all we want, and we will take good care of you. Thank you."

Enjoy your self-controlled meal, and give the server a decent tip.

2. Order a Doggie Bag

If your dining companion does not want to share, that is fine. Just say to your server: "I would like the blackened fish, baked potato and vegetable, but please split the entree in half. Put half of it in a take-out bag and the other half on my plate. Bring me the 'doggie bag' when you bring the check, please. Thank you."

3. Order Creatively

There is no law that says you must order a whole entree. Choose an appetizer, a starch and a salad for a well-balanced, low-fat meal. Look for starch side dishes such as pasta, rice, bread or hearty grain/legume soups. Or just say: "I would like the shrimp cocktail, a baked potato with A-1 sauce, and a salad with dressing on the side." Just because they are not combined in that way to make an entrée, if they are all on the menu somewhere, it is likely that the restaurant will be able to accommodate you. Do not feel like you are being "a pain"...you are the one paying for it, for pete's sake!

4. Stay Alert

Keep the bread basket on the other side of the table, or take your one piece and then tell the server that you are finished with it. Do not put yourself in a compromising position by letting it sit in front of you for the whole meal. The temptation is too much.

Beware of fatty appetizers with mayonnaise or cream sauces. Most dishes with cream sauces tend to be fattening. If you really want alcohol, choose wine or a light beer. Better yet, order soda water with a twist of lime. Order fresh fruit or sherbet for dessert, split a dessert, or go without dessert. A Good Guideline to Remember: Refrain from having both alcohol and dessert in the same meal. If you must have one, choose one or the other. Another Good Guideline: Choose bottled sauces over butter and sour cream. Go for the flavor, not the fat.

Asking for What You Want

Dining out on your own nutritional terms requires an assertive "this-is-what-I-want" attitude. Be direct but polite. Servers will cooperate if you say "please" and "thank you." Now, most restaurants have a low-calorie dressing available, vegetarian options or heart-healthy options. These days, restaurants are more open to the customer ordering less food. In many places, you can request the entrée as an appetizer portion. Then, you could have a salad and an appetizer *(smaller portions)* with the same entree taste. Ask them to charge you accordingly. Say "please" and "thank you." You CAN learn to be assertive with food.

What do you do, after eight perfect days of tournament dieting, when you are offered a delicious-looking piece of chocolate cake? Is it offered by your well-meaning mother-in-law who does not take "no" for an answer? Does your tenacity, will and strength of character crumble or do you rise up with an "I appreciate the offer, but no thank you"?

Most of us who have a tough time dealing with food control find it difficult to remain in control because of the fact that we never have learned to be assertive. "Oh, Erin, try just a little piece of my rum raisin soufflé, I made it especially for you!" Or, you walk into the local pizza shop and while ordering a medium pizza, the counter person says, "Well today, you can have two medium pizzas for the price of one! Don't you want two?" Sure I want two – I want three – but I only need to eat one and that's even sharing it with my vacuum-mouthed brother who can consume a pizza for breakfast.

Learning to be assertive when ordering a meal, or requesting only a portion of whatever someone else wants you to eat, can be a kind of self-actualization. Get what you need and not what someone else wants you to have, even if it is with the best of intentions. Of course, you must also be aware of those friends and family members who may try to throw you "off course" due to jealousy. They may see you losing weight, get concerned that soon you will look better than them, and try to offer you more food or convince you that you don't really need to be doing this. This phenomenon is more common than one might think.

So, let's practice: You are at a restaurant. The last time you ate there, you overdid it. Having learned that less is best, you have a new opportunity, so you order a salad with a shrimp cocktail and a baked potato...a small one with Worcestershire sauce instead of butter.

The waiter, looking you straight in the eye and through to your wallet asks, "Is that all?" You think his real meaning is, "Ok, cheapo. Can't come up with the bucks for a complete dinner, huh?" But you remain steadfast. "Yes, that is all I care for, thanks." Whew, got through that!

Good for you. You have made your decision and have stood by it. In an issue of American Health Magazine, the head chef of Commander's Palace, a five-star New Orleans restaurant, stated, "If a customer doesn't quite want what we offer on the menu, he/she can ask for something specific and we'll try to accommodate."

A real surprise comment from a busy chef, yet people need to learn to ask nicely and firmly, and say thank you. Be appreciative, be firm, and don't accept what you really don't want. Ask and you will probably receive. If you try it once or twice at each new place you go, you will find out which restaurants are more accommodating than others, and you can then choose to bring your business there.

Eating Out Responsibly

Remember, you can eat out at almost any restaurant if you make the right choices and control your portions responsibly, as with the above methods. Never go to a restaurant when you are extremely hungry. DANGER LURKS when your feel you are starving, and control is difficult. You will probably "blow it" while ordering or dine on the whole basket of bread while waiting for your meal to arrive.

Do you recall the last time you went to a restaurant really hungry, and you ordered a salad, appetizer and an entrée? And when the entrée finally arrived, you really did not even want it, but since you ordered it, you felt like you had to eat it anyway?

After finishing your meal and leaving the restaurant, you remarked to your spouse or dinner companion, "Why the heck *(optional words can be inserted)* did I do that? I ate way too much!" And, guess what? You could have split your favorite dessert, but no, you had to have it by yourself!

Fast Food Restaurants

There are numerous fast food choices with lower-fat options. Usually a grilled chicken sandwich without mayo or sauce is acceptable. The "without mayo or sauce" part of it is really important. Many fast food restaurants now have websites on which you can look up the fat, calories, and sodium content of foods on their menu. You may notice that some menu items have totally different values for "with sauce" versus "without sauce". This is because some of the sauces can add a significant amount of "hidden" calories that you are not likely to think about.

The burger joints are a challenge. One idea is to ask for a cheeseburger, but "hold" the burger, resulting in a cheese sandwich on a bun. Add lettuce, tomato, onion, pickles and a low-fat condiment *(mustard or ketchup)*, and you're OK. Some places call it "the vegetarian." Some places have now added veggie burgers to their menus. If you are not open to either of these options and must have an occasional burger, at least go for the smallest burger they have *(the "Jr. Hamburger" or whatever it may be called)* and order it without cheese. This way, you can get the taste you want but not the hundreds of additional calories that come along with the larger hamburgers and cheeseburgers.

Specific Suggestions for Eating at Fast Food Restaurants:

Always drink water or diet soda *(if need be)*, plan ahead, and stay in control!

Wendy's

1. Baked potato and a 1/2 order of chili
2. Baked potato with sour cream *(and broccoli?)* and taco sauce, plus a salad with lite dressing
3. "Vegetarian" cheeseburger without the burger but with all the toppings, hold the mayo
4. Grilled chicken sandwich
   Note: When ordering Mandarin or special salads, ask for lite dressing.

Chick-fil-A

1. Grilled chicken Snadwich or Salad
   Note: Ask for lite dressing.

Subway *(The overall best "fast food" restaurant in the land)*

1. Create your own low-fat sub, on whole wheat, with light sauces *(no mayo)*
2. A Veggie Delite Sub
3. On the side: get baked chips or ask for pickles 6.
4. NOT THE TUNA SUB! It has 19 grams of fat.
   Note: Subway does a great job at putting the nutritional information of each of their subs on display. Check it out to really get a sense of which ones are lower in fat. Also remember to use mustard or vinegar instead of mayo.

Burger King

Now offers baked potato, salads and a veggie burger.

MacDonald's

Not Much! Possibly a Chef's Salad, *but ask for light dressing* Yogurt Parfait

Arby's

1. Grilled chicken sandwich
2. Lite roast beef sandwich

Taco Bell

1. 1 bean burrito
2. 1 bean or chicken tostada
   Be aware of sour cream or guacamole.

Most fast food restaurants now post nutritional information on their websites. Check it out before you go, in order to have a head start on what are good nutritional choices.

General Recommendations

Beware of "Value Meals" which offer an economic incentive to stuff your gut! A Burger King Double Whopper Value Meal ranges from 1,600 to 2,100 calories depending on the size of the soft drink and fries. That is a LONG way from healthy.

Another general recommendation: DON'T GO TO ANY hamburger joints, fried chicken take-outs, Chinese buffets, or any "All You Can Eat" restaurants. You force yourself to make better choices when you give yourself better options to choose from. You can take control by not going to those places in the first place.

Don't Let "All You Can Eat" Bite You in the Tush

Probably the most dangerous place to eat, particularly when watching your weight, is the well-known "all-you-can-eat" buffet. Yes, I know there are some tasty buffets out there...Chinese, barbecue, Thai, or that traditional weekend Brunch buffet *(with mounds of glistening scrambled eggs, links of sausage, and pancakes)*. Have you ever watched horses eating around a trough?

Picture this: It is lunchtime, you are cruising around in your chariot, and your stomach grabs the wheel as you drive past the "All You Can Eat for $4.95" sign. What a deal! Where else can you spend so little and get so much! You park, get a table, get a plate and dig in. And you keep thinking, "Boy, am I saving money by eating here." Then, you feel like you really should eat all you can, to get the biggest "bang for your buck." Your mind can justify almost anything, but is this really saving?

With weight loss programs, you can pay a company $25 to get rid of the one lousy pound you added with that $4.95 "All You Can Eat" meal. Is it worth it? No! Hopefully you can spend your cash more wisely, putting meals and money into perspective. Think before you act, and you will make better decisions. For your one "splurge meal" of the week, wouldn't you rather eat at your favorite restaurant than at the $4.95 buffet?! Although I strongly recommend that anyone trying to lose weight stay FAR away from "food bars" or buffets, if you do happen to find yourself there, here are a few important tips to help you stay in control of your eating:

1) I know a rather large, good-natured, intelligent fellow who is known in some circles as the "Bane of the Buffet." He is the guy in front of you in line who leaves nothing in his wake. So get behind him and you'll have slim pickings, if anything. Just kidding.

Okay, now for the real tips:

1) A more practical idea is to peruse the buffet first withOUT a plate in hand. Make a mental note of the best-looking foods that aren't too fattening and then get in line with your plan in mind. Oh yes, and then follow your plan!

2) Get more of the low-fat food and only a little of the high-fat food. Fill half of your plate with different kinds of vegetables. Plus, get a salad.

3) Eat your salad first and eat your meal slowly.

4) Drink WATER *(or diet soda or unsweet tea, if necessary)* and lots of it. You really do not want to risk getting additional unnecessary calories from both the food AND the drink. Make it a point to drink half a glass of water before you go up to the buffet and the other half a glass within the first five minutes of your meal *(then refill and continue drinking normally)*. This way, at least some of your stomach will be full with water instead of with food.

5) Remember, you do not have to go back and get more. You will have still gotten your money's worth! The person that eats the most for the least is NOT the winner. So really think to yourself: "When is the last time I left a buffet meal and felt satisfied but not stuffed?" Never? Unless you can truly control yourself, a buffet is the WORST deal in town.

"Traveling is When I Blow My Diet"

Jeff, a close friend and attorney, once told me, "Freddy, traveling is when I blow my diet." With a little planning, it does not have to be so.

By Car

You are going on a trip – business or pleasure – and you have four hours of driving ahead of you. You leave at noon. In your rush to "get out of Dodge," you jump into the car, remembering to pack your toothbrush, but forgetting to eat lunch. By 2 p.m., hunger sets in. The need for a feeding frenzy overtakes reason as the "Greasy Spoon Emporium" comes into sight. You enter, the smells seduce you, and you quickly order without even thinking about it...the wrong foods and too much of it. You wind up back in the car uncomfortably stuffed and knowing the "Greasy Spoon Emporium" was a bad decision.

What should you do to avoid this situation? Before you leave town, have a reasonable, starched-based meal to sustain your blood sugar. Then, pack a cooler with water or diet sodas and some low-calorie snacks. Some tasty ones to try are: Quakes *(by Quaker)* Mini Flavored Rice Cakes *(cheddar cheese is my favorite)* and pretzels. Fruit, such as an apple, banana, or grapes, is always a good idea. Or make your own trail mix with popcorn, nuts, cereal, and dried fruit *(in individual small plastic bags to help portion control, as opposed to one big one)*. Make sure you do not start snacking until you are at least halfway there.

If you do stop to eat on the road, remember that most fast food restaurants offer a few lower-calorie choices. Do not just pull into the first restaurant you see. Think about what they offer before you commit. With a little thought, you could end up with a baked potato or grilled chicken instead of a cheeseburger or some fried whatever. If you know you are going to *(or can)* stop along the way, pack a picnic lunch. It could be as simple as a sandwich, piece of fruit, and a bottle of water. You will save money and enjoy a more controlled alternative. Many rest stops have nice picnic areas, some in wooded settings.

If you are driving longer distances, a walk before or during a long drive will help prevent fluid retention in your ankles and legs.

By Plane

Most of us agree that airplane food leaves a lot to be desired. Nowadays, you are lucky to get pretzels or crackers, unless you are flying internationally.

If you are making a quick trip on an in-state "puddle-jumper," stop by your favorite local sandwich shop on your way to the airport *(call ahead if you are in a hurry, so it is ready when you arrive)* and bring your lunch on-board. Now you can pass on the fat-filled honey roasted peanuts. You will be in total control and feeling good.

Too often, when you do have the time to sit and eat in an airport, you need to bring your banker or first born child as collateral *(the prices are so high)*. But now, many snack shops carry yogurt, cereal and a limited fruit selection. That is enough for a quick, satisfying, reasonably priced, and moderate-calorie meal.

If you do have to have a "treat"... I recall racing through the Atlanta airport, hurrying past numerous ice cream shops and hot dog stands before the familiar odor of fresh popcorn hit me. Ahhhh, my low-calorie travel alternative! The only problem with fresh popcorn on a plane is that people stare at you feverishly, with their eyes asking, "Where's mine?!" Another option is frozen yogurt. Get the low-fat kind.

By Boat

If you are talking about one of the big cruise ships that travel to the Bahamas or wherever, you are in for a major marathon feast. I have had clients who lost weight before a cruise simply because they expected to put the lost pounds back on, plus more, before the end of the cruise!

I have even heard of a prize for the couple that gains the most weight during the cruise! Can you imagine? If you don't want to gain, remember that the ship as well as any ports of call, are certainly large enough for a few walks each day.

(P.S. You don't have to eat all five courses for dinner every night.)

By Train

Here again, pack a healthy low-fat, nutritious snack or small meal. You can usually get a bottled water or diet drink on board. Do not expect the Orient Express dining, as imagined and portrayed in old movies. There will probably not be many *(if any)* healthy options on board, so it is best to bring something.

By Hot-Air Balloon

Eat and drink after you touch down, not during. The thrill and food don't mix.

Healthy Cooking Made Easy

Easy Portion Control
(Drum roll, please...)

Here are three good methods to help you control portions, in the beginning of the program or whenever you are having some difficulty. For easier portion control, these suggestions are best used as supper options because normally supper is the most difficult meal to control amounts.

1) The Frozen Meal and Salad

As mentioned earlier, there are numerous good-tasting, good for you, low-calorie, low-fat frozen meal options amidst the many "Hungry Man" varieties. Try Amy's, Healthy Choice, Lean Cuisine, Kashi, or Weight Watchers brands. Beware of Stouffers regular frozen meals; they are very dense in fat calories. Generally speaking, find a frozen meal that contains less than 10 grams of fat and that is 350 calories or less. Also, beware that the sodium content of these meals can be very high. Your RDA *(Recommended Daily Allowance)* for salt is 2400 mg *(1 tsp)* daily. If you read a frozen meal label that lists 690 mg of sodium, you might think it is high in sodium, but it really isn't too bad. Just be aware and read the nutritional content *(and refrain from adding salt to meals, in general)*. Look at the serving size and be sure that it is one serving and not two.

2) Soup and Salad

This traditional combo is a great way to control amounts, especially in the winter months. You definitely want to go for a hearty soup, not some thin broth chicken noodle soup, unless you embellish it *(bulk it up)* yourself. Try adding 1/2 cup of brown rice or 1/2 cup of canned *(washed and drained)* beans to make any soup thicker, as well as higher in fiber. Adding extra veggies is also always a good idea that will make your meal more nutritious.

One bowl or two cups of soup, along with a large mixed green salad, can be a wonderfully filling and healthy meal. Progresso, Health Valley, Amy's and Healthy Choice are reliable, hearty soup producers. Look for low-sodium options whenever possible *(the biggest problem with canned soups is that they tend to be really high in sodium)*. Alessi brand is good for a base. For a heartier soup, add peas, beans, brown rice, wild rice or noodles. Also, don't be shy about adding more flavors, such as light soy sauce, hot sauce, A-1, or even barbecue sauce. When you serve it, have a variety of sauces available to "doctor it up," as well as extra herbs *(oregano, basil, black pepper)*. Being creative with food does not have to be complicated. This is also a good option for when it is your turn to cook dinner and you want "an easy way out!"

3) A Shake for Supper

Have a Meal Replacement Shake as supper occasionally. Today, there are numerous quick, blended shakes, some already mixed and ready-to-go in a can, but I really recommend creating your own.

The Recipe:

6 oz. skim milk

½ large banana or 1 small banana *(try freezing ahead of time)* or other fruit

6 or more ice cubes

2 Tbsp. *(about 150 calories)* of whey or soy-based shake powder – OR - peanut butter

Note: You do not want a shake powder that is primarily protein. The best for the kidneys would be carbohydrate-based powders *(malts, dextran primarily, some sugar, and maybe 10-15 grams of protein)*. Some products such as: Twin Labs, Nature's Plus and Medibase are excellent.

Make a salad to go along with it. This way, you will get your veggies and also feel like you are eating more. The meal replacement shake for supper idea is a good way to control portions. It should fill you up; however, I recommend planning something to do right after the shake, in case it takes some time for your stomach to feel satisfied. Go to a movie or bookstore. Get out or have a project going on right after your "supper shake." This will prevent you from continuing to think about food and "grazing" in the kitchen.

Short-Order Cooking Made Shorter

Who has got the time to cook anything, let alone a healthy, low-fat, good-tasting meal? You do! Here's how. First, I highly recommend "batch cooking," which involves planning, shopping and then cooking larger *(i.e. large enough for more than one meal)* quantities of food to be refrigerated. The pre-cooked food will be available to then mix and match into convenient meals.

Note: If you "batch cook" the basics, such as: brown rice, new potatoes, noodles – preferably whole-grain, beans *(limas, butter beans)*, chicken breasts, etc., and keep them in small plastic containers in the fridge *(such that each container holds just enough for one meal serving)*, you will then have a food-control system. Additionally, keeping canned beans/peas and hearty, healthy soups on hand to be used as a basis for a meal is an excellent idea for healthy convenience.

How To Cook Brown Rice: *(makes 3 cups of cooked rice)*

Bring 2 cups of water to a boil. Add 1 cup of brown rice; then turn down heat to a simmer *("Low")*. Cover and cook for 45 minutes *(set the timer so you will know)*. DON'T STIR! When the timer goes off after 40-45 minutes, stick a fork straight in until it touches the bottom of the pot, then push a little of the rice aside to see if there is any water still in the pot. If so, cook a few more minutes. As soon as there is no moisture, take the pot off the burner and "fluff" the rice with a fork so it does not stick to the pot. Believe me – this is not complicated – it is just something you have to do once or twice, and then you will know how to do it. The biggest key is not stirring the rice. You want it to be fluffy, not mushy.

For additional flavor, try substituting low-sodium vegetable or chicken broth for half of the water, or adding a cube or two of low-sodium vegetable or chicken bouillon when water begins to boil. Or add herbs such as rosemary or oregano and a little olive oil.

Cooking Tofu

"Weird!" "Not in my lifetime!" "Are you crazy?" Oh, the comments! But you can bake it, grill it, barbeque it, stir-fry it, and blend it in a multitude of ways. The continent that brought us Honda cars and Sony televisions has also brought us TOFU, the hamburger of Asia. Tofu, a staple in Asia for 2,000 years, is an easy to digest, somewhat bland food with a similar texture to cheese. It pleasantly picks up the flavor of whatever you cook with it. It is made from soybean curd and can be substituted in many dishes in place of meat. Tofu is a complete source of protein and contains no animal fat or cholesterol, few calories and an excellent source of iron and Vitamin B.

A simple way to use tofu is to just substitute tofu for chicken. You can cut up tofu in small cubes or slice it in different sizes. Some people say tofu has no "real" flavor of its own. This is somewhat true, but that can really be a pro instead of a con. Why? Because it picks up the flavor of whatever you cook it in or pour over it. Like barbeque sauce? You can have barbeque tofu! Have a favorite marinade? It will soak it up better than any meat.

Blocks of refrigerated tofu from your grocery store come in silken, soft, firm or extra firm varieties or even as tofu crumbles. The firm and extra firm are great for stir-fry, baking, or barbeque. DO NOT accidentally buy silken or soft *(the kind used in miso soup)* and try to use it in a stir-fry, because you will end up with mush and never try tofu again. Just follow the simple directions or recipes on the package. BE SURE to use a kitchen towel or many paper towels and press as much water out of it as possible BEFORE you cook it, to make it less watery and allow it to soak up more of your sauce. Tofu crumbles are a wonderful substitute for meat in spaghetti sauce, Sloppy Joes, meatballs, chili, and especially tacos. They are a great first way to try tofu. Make spaghetti "meat" sauce like you normally do or even by the pre-made taco meat seasoning and use the tofu crumbles instead *(p.s. - this is a good way to trick a reluctant spouse into eating it)*. Try it, you'll like it dahling! ...I hope.

Stir-Frying Tofu: Frequently, at home, we stir-fry tofu in a combination of several of the following. Feel free to pick and choose:

Olive oil	Honey
Soy sauce	Sesame seeds
(use the low-sodium kind)	A-1 Sauce
Garlic, minced	Worcestershire sauce
Ginger, minced	Barbecue sauce
(Lite) salt and pepper	Peanut sauce

Chop tofu into small cubes or strips. Add the rest of the ingredients. Cook over medium heat in a skillet that has been coated with vegetable cooking spray or olive oil. Spread out cubes and let cook. Flip over and cook for the same time on the other sides. Limit stirring or flipping to reduce breakage, but don't let it stick to the pan. Tofu absorbs the flavors it is cooked in. It is best cooked slowly and in my opinion, well done, so it is firm. Serve with brown rice and steamed veggies.

An example tofu recipe follows. Please feel free to look more up! You will be amazed at how much you can do with tofu – a cheap and healthy food and meat substitute.

Tofu Loaf *(a healthy alternative to the traditional Meat Loaf)*

Preheat oven to 350° F

1 ½ lbs. tofu, mashed
⅓ cup ketchup
⅓ cup soy sauce
2 Tbsp. Dijon mustard
½ cup parsley, chopped
¼ tsp. black pepper
1 medium onion, chopped fine
¼ t. Garlic powder
1 cup whole grain bread crumbs, rolled oats, or cornflakes, crushed

Mix all ingredients together. Put ¼ oil in a loaf pan, then press the mixture into the pan. Bake for about 1 hour. Let cool 10-15 minutes before trying to remove from pan. Garnish with ketchup and parsley. Also good sliced and sautéed for sandwiches the next day.

Serves 6-8. Makes one loaf pan.

Per Serving: Calories: 226, Protein: 10 grams, Fat: 13 grams, Carbohydrates: 18 grams.

Cookbooks Galore!

There are many excellent cookbooks available with low-fat, healthy, low-calorie recipes. Here are a few:

Lean and Luscious by Bobbie Hinman and Millie Snyder

Meals on the Move (Rush Hour Recipes) by Holly Berkowitz Clegg

Pacific Grilling: Recipes from the Fire from Baja to the Pacific Northwest by Denis Kelly

The Everything Slow Cooker Cookbook by Margaret Kaeter

Bean Banquets from Boston to Bombay by Patricia Gregory

The Moosewood cookbooks by Mollie Katzen, Pam Krauss

Secrets of Good-Carb, Low-Carb Living by Sandra Woodruff, R.D.

The Good Carb Cookbook by Sandra Woodruff, R.D.

Tofu Cookery by Louise Hagler

Informative Magazines

Here are some magazines that also can help you out:

Nutrition Action Health Letter, by Center for Science in the Public Interest

Vegetarian Times

Environmental Nutrition: The Newsletter of Food, Nutrition, and Health

Eating Well: Where Good Taste Meets Good Health

Healthy Food Staples to Keep on Hand

Vegetable oils and sprays – OLIVE OIL IS THE BEST

Rice – preferably brown

Bread – whole wheat, multigrain

Bagels – whole-grain, multigrain or oat bran

Pasta – white and whole wheat

Tomato sauces, cubed or strained

Spices, salt substitutes

Fruits – bananas, grapes, apples, oranges, peaches *(frozen bananas to use in blended shakes and smoothies)*

Vegetables – fresh, frozen, or canned *(low-sodium variety)*

Potatoes – sweet *(better)* and white *(baking, red or new potatoes)*

Chicken breasts

Beans and peas – frozen or canned

Fish – salmon, tuna, sardines

Soups – hearty ones such as Progresso, Amy's, Health Valley *(low-sodium variety, if possible)*

Frozen meals – Amy's, Healthy Choice, Lean Cuisine, Kashi, Weight Watchers

Sauces – A-1, PickAPeppa, Worcestershire, Soy, and BBQ sauces, Crystal Hot Sauce

"I Can't Believe It's Not Butter" Spray Margarine

Curry Paste *(Patak brand)*

Most foods, no matter how bland, can be made to taste good, by using various sauces for flavoring.

Example food & sauce combinations:

rice	soy sauce, barbeque sauce, Worcestershire sauce *(contains anchovies, so Vegans Beware)*, spray margarine
pasta	tomato sauce, garlic and spray margarine, light olive oil and spices
beans *(such as kidney, limas, navy)*	barbecue sauce, soy sauce, Crystal Louisiana Hot Sauce
potatoes	salsa, Worcestershire sauce, ketchup, light sour cream, soups
vegetables	spray olive oil, spray margarine, lemon pepper, soups, soy sauce, Louisiana hot or mild sauces

Recipes for Healthy Living

There are numerous excellent cookbooks available on healthy, low-fat cooking. Open most newspapers to the food and/or health sections to find various recipes as well. Here are a few of my most useful "KISS" *(Keep It Simple, Stupid)* recipes for nights when you do not really feel like "cooking," but could manage taking 30 minutes or less to "put something together."

Simple Recipes

1. "SOUP DU JOUR" *(Soup of the Day)*

A) 1 can lentil soup *(try Progresso's or Amy's brands)*
2 cups steamed/cooked potatoes, carrots, celery, onions and Brussels sprouts *(or not)*
1 t. curry powder *(if you like that taste, if not, use other flavoring)*
1 t. chopped garlic

Just mix and simmer for 5 minutes. Serve with a large green salad. ENJOY!

B) 1 can Condensed Potato Soup
2 cups skim milk or water
2 cups steamed/cooked potatoes, carrots and broccoli
1 cup navy or cannelloni beans
1 tablespoon chopped garlic
2 bay leaves

Mix all ingredients together and simmer for 5 minutes. Serve with green salad.

Note: You can do the same with Split Pea soup, Tomato soup, "Lite" Minestrone soup, etc. Add your desired combination of vegetables, pasta, potato or rice to make a hearty meal.

2. VEGGIE BURGER

Try varieties such as Garden Burger, Morning Star, or Boca Burgers. They all have multiple varieties, so keep trying different versions until you find one that you like. Garden Burger offer varieties such as: Flame Grilled (*most similar to a regular meat burger*), The Original (*made with grains, cheese, and veggies*), Portabella, Sun-dried Tomato Basil (*has a pizza-type flavor*) or Black Bean Chipotle (*a little spicy*). If you are lactose-intolerant, look for the varieties that say "Vegan" on the box. Serve with vegetarian Bush Baked Beans or butter beans and a salad.

3. "SUCCOTASH" – southern goodness

Mix together and heat: tomatoes, onions, okra, corn, butter beans or lima beans. Flavor with: garlic, a little olive oil, 1 teaspoon cilantro and pepper, to taste.

4. BEAN BURRITOS

> ½ cup fat-free refried beans (*try El Paso or Rosarita brands*)
> 2 flour tortillas (*whole wheat is better*)
> Chopped tomatoes and green lettuce
> ½ oz. low-fat cheddar cheese (*per burrito*)
> Salsa and/or chopped jalapeño peppers (*if you like spicy*)

Spread half of the beans on one surface of each tortilla. Sprinkle with cheddar cheese and add tomatoes. Heat them for a few seconds in the microwave. Add lettuce. The salsa/jalapeño peppers are optional for spice and flavor. Fold lower end of tortilla to form bottom of burrito, then roll by thirds to finish.

5. BLACK-EYED PEAS AND BROWN RICE

Canned black-eyed peas are the most convenient *(rinse and drain first),* unless you have already "batch cooked" some dried black-eyed peas and have them waiting in the fridge for you. Brown rice takes approximately 45 minutes to cook, and the ratio of water to rice is usually 2:1. There are also quick-cooking varieties of brown rice that you can get, if need be. Flavor with brown mustard, pickle relish, onions, garlic, and spices, as desired. Have steamed vegetables on the side. If desired, find a whole-grain cornbread mix *(harder to find, but the brand Martha White now offers one that can be found in regular grocery stores)* and add a small can of corn to the mixture before baking.
NOTE: See the previous chapter on Healthy Cooking for instructions on cooking brown rice.

6. BLACK BEANS AND RICE

Basic but delicious Latin cuisine. Spice it up the way you like it! For a quick fix, use canned beans. Heat them up in a pot with diced onions, green peppers, and 1 tsp. minced garlic. Flavor them with oregano and salsa. Top with 1.2 oz. low-fat cheddar cheese or 1 tsp. low-fat sour cream and diced tomatoes. Remember that brown rice is better than white rice, because brown rice has more fiber, vitamins, and minerals. NOTE: See the previous chapter on Healthy Cooking for instructions on cooking brown rice.

7. THE "MEXICAN MIX UP"

Another version of the traditional black beans and rice. Mix up a can of Contadina "Pasta Ready" Chunky Tomatoes and canned corn with the black beans and rice.

8. VEGETARIAN "BEANS ON TOAST"

Use vegetarian fat-free baked beans with brown mustard over whole wheat bread. Add a green veggie.

9. THE CHILI POTATO

Use fat-free, meatless chili over a baked potato AND 1.2 oz. of low-fat cheddar cheese. Add a green veggie (*try steaming broccoli, chopping into little pieces, and mixing it in*).

10. PASTA FAGIOLI

This means "pasta and beans" in Italian and is a traditional meatless Italian dish. It was originally considered a peasant dish, because beans and pasta were both cheaply available, but is now served throughout the world. Add cannellini beans or navy beans to some type of small pasta (*preferably whole-grain*), and season with olive oil, garlic, minced onion (*optional*), and tomato sauce or Contadina Pasta Ready. Add additional spices (*oregano, basil*) as desired.

11. NEW POTATOES WITH GARBANZO/KIDNEY BEANS

Or, use any other type of beans or peas. Add 1-2 tsp. of Biryani curry paste or salsa. Microwave to warm.

Soups

From the following recipes, one bowl of soup *(any of these soups)* will equal approximately 300 to 350 calories and when paired with a green salad, would make an excellent complete meal. All beans/peas/lentils could be from the can, frozen, or cooked from scratch.

The following chili and soup recipes are for those of you who enjoy cooking.

For those just getting acquainted with making or eating entrées composed of beans and grains, this saucy chili is invariably a favorite:

Note: Stock - chicken, vegetable or beef could be added to any liquid.

BEAN AND VEGETABLE CHILI

2 tablespoons olive oil
1 large onion, chopped
1 medium red pepper, chopped
1 small zucchini squash, thinly sliced
1 cup cooked fresh or *(thawed)* frozen corn kernels
1 14 oz *(400 g)* can plum tomatoes with liquid, chopped
1 6 oz *(180 g)* can tomato paste
3 tablespoons soy sauce or tamari sauce
2 teaspoons chili powder, more or less to taste
1 teaspoon ground cumin
½ teaspoon ground coriander
½ teaspoon dried oregano
¼ teaspoon dried thyme
Cayenne pepper to taste, optional
2 ½ cups cooked or canned kidney or black beans *(about 1 cup dried, cooked following package directions)*
Pickled green chilies for garnish, optional
low-fat cheddar cheese for garnish, optional

Heat the oil in a very large skillet. When it is hot, add the onion and sauté over low to medium-low heat until the onion is translucent. Add the red pepper and sauté until it softens somewhat. Add the remaining ingredients, including the beans, and simmer over very low heat for at least 15 minutes, or longer to let the flavors mix, and stir occasionally. Serve in bowls garnished with a green chili and low-fat cheddar cheese, and even better, over brown rice.

Makes 4 to 6 servings.

WHITE BEAN & BLACK OLIVE SOUP

1. First, cook 1 cup dried white navy beans for 1½ hours. *(Canned beans are fine, just rinse them first)*
2. Then, assemble and sauté the following in medium pot:
   3 tablespoons olive oil
   3-4 cloves crushed garlic
   ½ cup chopped celery
   ½ cup chopped green pepper
   1 cup zucchini chunks
   ½ cup chopped carrots
   ½ teaspoon salt; pepper to taste
   1 teaspoon oregano
   1 ½ teaspoons basil
3. Add the following to the pot:
   4 cups low-sodium stock or water
   ½ cup sliced black olives
   3 oz. tomato paste
   Add the cooked white navy beans from above.
4. Simmer on low for 1/2 hour.
5. When serving, add the following:
   1 tablespoon lemon juice
   ¼ cup chopped parsley

KALE, CABBAGE AND WHITE BEAN SOUP

This soup is hearty, flavorful and very nutritious. This is a rather thick soup; if you prefer a thinner soup, just add some more water.

1 cup dried baby lima beans *(must be soaked for 8 hours or overnight) (may use canned or frozen)*

5 cups water

1 strip kombu *(type of sea vegetable)*, 6 inches long

1 ½ cups chopped onion

3 cups chopped kale

2 cups finely chopped cabbage

1 teaspoon savory

1-2 tablespoons lemon juice *(or to taste)*

¼ cup miso *(or to taste)* barley miso is good, as is yellow or white miso

1. Wash the lima beans and place them in a medium-sized bowl. Add enough water to cover, with about 1 ½ inches more water than beans, and soak for at least 8 hours.
2. Drain the soaked beans and place them in a large kettle with 5 cups of water. Cover the kettle and bring to a boil. Lower the heat and simmer the beans for about 1 hour or until tender.
3. Rinse the strip of kombu and put it in the kettle with the beans. Add the chopped onion, kale, cabbage and savory. Cover and simmer for about 1/2 hour more, or until the vegetables are tender.
4. Remove the kettle from the heat and add lemon juice and miso. Remove the kombu and either discard it or chop it into bite-sized pieces and return it to the soup. Mix well and serve with whole-grain bread.

Makes 4 to 6 servings.

VEGETABLE GUMBO

When used in a soup, diced okra loses its undesirable texture and becomes very delicious. This recipe makes a large kettle of soup; you may wish to cut in half.

½ cup barley
6 cups water or vegetable broth
1 large carrot, sliced
1½ cups chopped onion
3-4 cloves garlic, minced
1½ cups green beans, broken in ½ inch pieces
2 cups finely chopped white cabbage
3 bay leaves
3 cups canned tomatoes or finely chopped fresh tomatoes
2 tablespoons tamari, or to taste
1½ cups corn, cut off the cob
2 cups sliced okra
1 teaspoon basil
2-3 tablespoons olive oil *(optional)*

1. Wash the barley and place it in a large kettle with the 6 cups of water or vegetable stock. Cover and bring to a boil. Reduce heat and simmer for about 1 1/2 hours.
2. Add the carrot, onion, garlic, green beans, cabbage, bay leaves, tomatoes and tamari. Cover and simmer until the vegetables are almost tender.
3. Add the corn, okra, and basil. Simmer for about 15 minutes more, or until the okra is cooked.
4. Add the olive oil, if desired. If the soup is too thick for your taste, add some water or tomato juice. Add more tamari to taste, if you wish.

Makes 6 to 8 servings.

HOMEMADE VEGETABLE SOUP

1 ¾ cups peeled, cubed potatoes
1½ cups chopped onion
1 cup sliced carrot
1 cup sliced celery
½ teaspoon dried whole basil
¼ teaspoon dried whole thyme
2 bay leaves
2 *(13 ½-ounce)* cans, no-salt-added beef broth, undiluted
1 cup water
¼ cup no-salt-added tomato paste
3 *(14½-ounce)* cans, no-salt-added whole tomatoes,
    undrained
1 *(10-ounce)* package frozen whole kernel corn, thawed
1 *(10-ounce)* package frozen baby lima beans, thawed
1 *(10-ounce)* package frozen sliced okra, thawed

Combine the first 10 ingredients in a large Dutch oven *(or a large pot)*. Place tomatoes, in batches, in an electric blender. Blend tomatoes until smooth; add to broth mixture. Bring to a boil, then cover, reduce heat, and simmer for 30 minutes.

Add corn and lima beans to tomato mixture; bring to a boil. Cover, reduce heat, and simmer another 20 minutes, stirring occasionally. Add okra. Bring to a boil; reduce heat and simmer 5 minutes. Remove and discard bay leaves.
Makes 15 cups.

Nutritional Information: 145 calories *(3% from fat)* per 1 ½ cup serving. Fat = 0.5 grams. Protein = 6 grams. Carbohydrate = 31.1 grams Fiber = 4.2 grams. Cholesterol = 0 mg. Sodium = 84 mg.

ZUCCHINI AND TOMATO SOUP

2 cups coarsely shredded zucchini squash
2 *(8-ounce)* cans no-salt-added tomato sauce
1 ½ cups sliced fresh mushrooms
1 cup canned vegetable broth, undiluted
⅓ cup finely chopped onion
1 small clove garlic, minced
½ teaspoon dried whole basil
½ teaspoon dried whole oregano
1 *(14 ½-ounce)* can no-salt-added whole tomatoes,
   un-drained and diced
1 ½ teaspoons lemon juice
¼ teaspoon salt
⅛ teaspoon pepper
½ tablespoon freshly grated Parmesan cheese

Combine first 8 ingredients in a large saucepan; bring to a boil. Reduce heat and simmer, uncovered, 25 minutes or until zucchini and mushrooms are tender, stirring occasionally. Add tomato, lemon juice, salt, and pepper; cook until thoroughly heated. Ladle soup into individual bowls; sprinkle evenly with cheese.

MICROWAVE DIRECTIONS: Combine first 8 ingredients in a 3-quart casserole; cover with heavy-duty plastic wrap, and vent. Microwave on HIGH 18 minutes or until zucchini is tender, stirring after 9 minutes. Stir in tomato, lemon juice, salt and pepper. Microwave on HIGH 1 to 2 minutes or until mixture is thoroughly heated. Ladle soup into individual bowls; sprinkle evenly with cheese.

Makes 6 one-cup servings.

Nutritional Info: 68 calories *(13% from fat)* per each 1 cup serving. Fat = 1.3 grams. Protein = 3.4 grams. Carbohydrate = 12.6 grams. Fiber = 2.3 grams. Cholesterol = 1 mg. Sodium = 177 mg.

HERBED SPLIT PEA SOUP

½ pound dried split peas
3 *(10½ ounce)* cans low-sodium chicken broth, undiluted
¾ cup chopped onion
½ cup chopped carrot
½ teaspoon ground celery seeds
¼ teaspoon salt
¼ teaspoon dried whole marjoram, crushed
¼ teaspoon freshly ground pepper
⅛ teaspoon dried whole thyme
Fresh thyme sprigs *(optional)*

Sort and wash peas; place in a Dutch oven. Add broth and next 8 ingredients. Bring to a boil; cover, reduce heat, and simmer 1 hour or until peas are tender. Blend mixture in batches in an electric blender or food processor; process until smooth. Return puree to pot. Cook over medium heat just until thoroughly heated *(do not boil)*. Ladle soup into individual bowls. Garnish with fresh thyme sprigs, if desired.
Makes 5 one-cup servings.

Nutritional Info: 221 calories *(11% from fat)* per 1 cup serving. Fat = 2.8 grams. Protein = 17.3 grams. Carbohydrate= 33.2 grams. Fiber = 3.6 grams. Cholesterol = 9 mg. Sodium = 475 mg.

SUMMER SQUASH SOUP

Vegetable cooking spray
2 teaspoons reduced-calorie margarine
1 cup chopped onions
2 tablespoons chopped fresh parsley
1 ½ teaspoons minced fresh basil
1 ¾ pounds yellow squash, cut into ¼ inch slices

193

1 medium zucchini, cut into ¼ inch slices
1 cup canned vegetable broth, undiluted
½ teaspoon salt
⅛ teaspoon ground white pepper
1 cup skim milk
Chopped fresh chives *(optional)*

Coat a Dutch oven *(or large pot)* with vegetable cooking spray; add margarine. Place over medium-high heat until margarine melts. Add onion, parsley, and basil; sauté until onion is tender. Add yellow squash and next 4 ingredients; cover and cook over medium heat 15-20 minutes or until squash is tender, stirring occasionally. Add milk, stirring constantly.

Blend mixture, in batches, in an electric blender or food processor; process until smooth. Return puree to pot. Cook over medium heat just until thoroughly heated *(do not boil)*. Ladle soup into individual bowls. Garnish with chopped fresh chives, if desired.

Makes 5 one-cup servings.

Nutritional Info: 77 calories *(23% from fat)* per 1 cup serving. Fat = 2.0 grams. Protein = 4.5 grams. Carbohydrate = 11.9 grams. Fiber = 3.2 grams. Cholesterol = 1 mg. Sodium = 307 mg.

TOMATO BASIL SOUP

4 cups peeled, seeded, and chopped tomatoes
2 ½ cups no-salt-added tomato juice
1 cup coarsely chopped onion
¼ cup chopped fresh basil
2 cloves garlic, halved
½ teaspoon salt
¼ teaspoon ground white pepper

2 tablespoons reduced-calorie margarine
3 tablespoons all-purpose flour
1 ½ cups skim milk
Fresh basil leaves (optional)

Combine first 7 ingredients in an electric blender or food processor; process until smooth. Transfer mixture to a saucepan; bring to a boil. Cover, reduce heat, and simmer 10 minutes, stirring occasionally.

Melt margarine in a small heavy saucepan over medium heat; add flour, stirring until smooth. Cook 1 minute, stirring constantly. Gradually add milk. Cook stirring constantly, until thickened and bubbly. Gradually stir sauce mixture into tomato mixture. Cook over medium heat just until thoroughly heated *(do not boil)*. Ladle soup into individual bowls. Garnish with fresh basil leaves, if desired.

Makes 6 one-cup servings.

Nutritional Info: 114 calories (24% from fat) per 1 cup serving. Fat = 3.1 grams. Protein = 5.0 grams. Carbohydrate = 19.3 grams. Fiber = 2.6 grams. Cholesterol = 1 mg. Sodium = 287 mg.

Important News Articles

Wake Up, America!

The following excerpts of articles from newspapers and newsletters are presented here to enhance your awareness of what messages should be of concern to you.

FAST FOOD COMPANIES HELP KEEP CONSUMERS IN THE DARK

(excerpt)

By Neal D. Barnard of Knight Ridder Tribune:

When New York attorney Samuel Hirsch filed a lawsuit on behalf of overweight and diabetic children, alleging that McDonald's had contributed to their health problems, many people reacted with disgust. Whatever happened to personal responsibility? How could anyone not know that fast food is bad for you?

As Dr. William Castelli of the Framingham Heart Study used to say, "When you see the Golden Arches, you're probably on the road to the pearly gates." Everybody knows that, right?

Well, frankly, everyone does not know that. The fact is, many members of the public are thoroughly confused about what to eat and food industries are capitalizing on their ignorance. In July [2002], a New York Times Magazine cover story suggested that fatty foods are not the real culprit after all, despite abundant evidence to the contrary. The real cause of obesity, the article went on, was carbohydrates.

While that article was wildly inaccurate (Asians and vegetarians consume large amounts of carbohydrate and yet, are the thinnest people on the planet), a surprising number of intelligent readers continued to look skeptically at rice, potatoes and pasta, and started letting meat, cheese and fried foods off the hook.

Fatty foods seemed to gain another reprieve in news reports portraying the greasy and cholesterol-laden Atkins Diet as somehow healthful. These reports never explained that the diet causes no weight loss at all unless enough other foods are left off the plate to keep the overall calorie content down, and even then, it can spark calcium loss that could spell osteoporosis over the long run, not to mention the links between meaty diets and colon cancer and heart disease. When educated adults are befuddled by simple nutrition issues, how can we expect that children, who rank among the fast food chains' principal targets, to understand the factors that contribute to becoming overweight or acquiring type 2 diabetes or other conditions?

...Are you aware that grilled chicken has one of the highest levels of carcinogenic compounds of any food? Do you realize that the McDonald's fish sandwich is almost 50 percent fat and has more grams of fat than the chain's cheeseburger (and only 1 gram less than the quarter pounder)? Did you know that men who frequently consume milk products, such as the average milkshake, have higher prostate cancer risk than people who avoid milk?

Consumers can often reel off the health risks of smoking, but many have no clue when it comes to the health risks of unhealthy eating. Although some Americans have given up or cut down on red meat in recent years, they've ironically switched to chicken, which actually has about the same amount of cholesterol and plenty of other health risks.

...It should be said that some restaurant chains have begun to offer healthful choices, such as Burger King's BK veggie burger, Taco Bell's bean burrito or the salad bars and baked potato bars offered elsewhere. But we have a very long way to go. Distasteful as litigation may be, if

197

lawsuits push industry to offer better products and to educate consumers about the links between diet and disease, that is all for the better.

DRUGS IN OUR FOOD: A NATIONAL SECURITY ISSUE? [22]

(excerpt)

By Arianna Huffington of the Tribune Media Services, February 14, 2002:

Would you like a side of fries with that cruise missile?

In a speech at a cattle industry convention last week, the president added yet another item to the ever-expanding list of things essential to our national security: food.

..."It's in our national security interests that we be able to feed ourselves," George Bush told the red meat meeting. "This nation has got to eat." That's very true, Mr. President. Second grade clearly wasn't wasted on you! But does the menu have to include beef brimming with growth-enhancing steroids and chicken laced with heavy-duty antibiotics? I realize that the Rancher-in-Chief has an affinity for guys wearing Stetsons, but listening to him sing the praises of "American's healthy beef" was, if you'll excuse me, hard to swallow.

Since the 1950s, some American farmers have been fattening their cattle with growth hormones...Fully two-thirds of this country's 36 million beef cattle are currently on the juice. Hormones are also regularly used to make cows more fertile and increase the amount of milk they produce.

Fears about the health hazards posed by the chronic use of these drugs led the European Union in 1989 to ban the importation of all hormone-treated meat. But, instead of taking these concerns to heart and reexamining U.S. policy, both the Clinton and Bush administrations imposed retaliatory trade sanctions against the EU.

And the contamination goes beyond the meat itself. Giant cattle feed lots and factory hog farms are generating massive manure runoffs that are responsible for the polluting of 60,000 miles of rivers and streams, putting our drinking water at risk and killing millions of fish. So while Tom Ridge is busy trying to figure out how to keep terrorists from slipping unwanted chemicals into your food and water, the meat industry is doing just that on a daily basis, with the government's cheerful backing.

And the situation isn't any more mouth-watering on the poultry portion of the menu. Chickens, cooped up in jam-packed factory feed lots, are routinely dosed with antibiotics just to help them survive the horrendous living conditions. Of the 26.6 million pounds of antibiotics stuffed down the throats of animals every year, only two million are used for treating specific illnesses. No wonder Colonel Sanders was always so diligent about keeping his vaunted recipe a secret.

As a result of this pervasive use of antibiotics, scientists have documented an alarming, though not surprising, increase in drug-resistant bacteria in humans, particularly since 1995, when the FDA, over the protests of the Centers for Disease Control, allowed the poultry industry to begin giving chickens a new class of powerful antibiotics that include Cipro.

...A number of poultry producers, responding to public pressure, have recently promised to substantially cut back on the antibiotics they feed healthy chickens. On the other hand, since our leaders in Washington, who were fed close to $9 million in campaign donations by the meat and dairy industries in the 2000 election cycle, don't require farmers to keep track of how much of the stuff they use, we'll apparently just have to take their word for it...

WEIGHING THE COST OF OBESITY:
Treating Obesity as a Disease Could Take Billions, But Save Lives, Money in the Long Run [23]

(excerpt)

By Nanci Hellmich of *USA Today*, January 20, 2002:

Is being fat an illness that should be covered by insurance? It's true that obesity contributes to diabetes, heart disease, arthritis and some types of cancer. But is obesity, on its own, a disease? That's a question that experts and advocacy groups are asking Americans to consider. And the answer is likely to be costly.

Obesity is a growing problem in this country - about 26%, or about 54 million adults are obese, roughly 30 or more pounds over a healthy weight, and about 300,000 deaths a year are attributed to obesity. The surgeon general recently issued a call to action to reduce those numbers, and he suggested talking about classifying obesity as a disease that would qualify for reimbursement.

Such a move could open the door for more doctors' visits, nutrition counseling and diet drugs to be covered. No one knows the exact costs, but estimates suggest it could be several billion dollars a year.

Right now, some health insurers cover obesity treatments, but it's far from universal. Physicians often don't tackle patients' weight problems during office visits because they won't get reimbursed for their time. And in many cases, prescription diet drugs aren't covered.

The nation's leading obesity organizations are pushing to change that. They say obesity is a disease that needs medical intervention and should be covered by insurance, HMOs, Medicare and Medicaid. They argue that more people would seek help if it was covered, and they say that even modest weight loss of as little as 5% produces health benefits such as lowering blood pressure and blood sugar and improving cholesterol levels. And they argue that those changes may save health care costs in the long run.

...If obesity isn't covered, "people will continue to get bigger and sicker," says Charles Billington, associate director of the Minnesota Obesity Center in Minneapolis.

Morgan Downey, executive director of the American Obesity Association, an advocacy group working to promote public policies on obesity, says: "Obesity is the engine that is driving a lot of diseases - heart disease, diabetes, hypertension, arthritis. We're paying for those diseases, but not contributing nearly enough to deal with the underlying cause, and that just doesn't make sense."

MORE NAGGING WON'T LEAD TO A SLIMMER AMERICA

(excerpt)

By Edward Achorn of Knight Ridder Tribune

The experts have issued their millionth warning about obesity, oddly timed, right before Christmas and our seasonal mandatory revels. Or maybe not so oddly timed, since the experts seem to believe that mindless, churlish hectoring will get us to change our ways.

Fat chance.

Surgeon General David Satcher took his shot, with his call on schools, communities and industries to fight fat. Americans are eating themselves to an early death at a rate of 300,000 a year, and Dr. Satcher estimates two of three Americans are now overweight, with the number rising. Even 13 percent of youngsters are now overweight, and Type II diabetes, once confined to adults, afflicts children as young as 10.

Part of the problem, the surgeon general argues, is intake of super-size fast foods. Some 40 percent of the American food budget is now spent eating (or taking) out. We are gross in more ways than one. Dr. Satcher wishes that schools would serve less fattening meals and restrict student access to soda machines; that employers would give employees time to exercise; and that communities would lay out more walking *trails. His critics think he stopped short: that he should have advocated greater public subsidies for fresh fruit and vegetables, and constructing gymnasiums in "high-risk" neighborhoods, where the propensity to bloat is especially great.*

...In truth, for all our fond wishes and public-service announcements, we won't see any changes soon. Americans will keep getting fatter. Ironically, that is, in part, because we do not care about food all that much. It's in the culture. The French linger over a meal for hours, savoring flavor, in conversation and choking clouds of cigarette smoke. We want our food abundant and fast, and then we rush off to do other things, like make money or rule the world.

And this is nothing new. Many 19th century European visitors were appalled by the way Americans silently wolfed down their food. Charles Dickens, who toured the United States in 1842, described such a scene in his novel Martin Chuzzlewit: "All the knives and forks were working away at a rate that was quite alarming; very few words were spoken; and everybody seemed to eat his utmost in self-defense, as if a famine were expected. Great heaps of indigestible matter melted away as ice before the sun." Imagine if Dickens had visited Burger King!...

FOOD MARKETING MADNESS

"Don't just stand there! Eat something!" urge the ads for granola bars at bus stops in downtown areas across the country, as if Americans need any more encouragement to eat. From television to T-shirts, from Internet banner ads to billboards, we're exposed to hundreds of messages every day to buy and eat more.

"We're bombarded incessantly by sophisticated psychological manipulations to convince us to eat junk food, drink alcohol, smoke tobacco, and watch violent entertainment," says Gary Ruskin, director of Commercial Alert, a nonprofit group in Washington, D.C., that opposes excesses in commercialism, advertising, and marketing.

Because corporations don't respect boundaries, he adds, "We fear they'll turn our homes into showrooms for pitchmen, our schools into amphitheaters for marketing, and our national parks into billboard showcases."

And children are now becoming prime targets. "Corporations used to respect the fact that children are precious beings to be nurtured," says Ruskin. "Now, under pressure to increase profits, many corporations see kids as economic resources to be exploited, like raw timber or bauxite."

"Many parents fear that corporations will turn our kids into smoking, drinking, violence-loving, obese addicts," he adds. Even schools don't offer refuge. More than 12,000 of them subscribe to Channel One, a daily commercial television news program broadcast by satellite. "These schools force their children to sit and watch commercials for fast foods and soft drinks, the very kinds of foods that are making them fatter," says Ruskin. And not just fatter. Ads push foods like burgers, fries, pizza, and ice cream, all prepping our kids and teens for a lifetime of grid-locked arteries and steadily rising blood pressure.

"There's been such a dramatic increase in advertising and corporate power over the past three decades that many of us have a growing sense that the relentless creep of commercialism threatens much of what makes life worth living," says Ruskin.

Food marketing and advertising have increased dramatically in recent years. From 1988 through 1999, the number of dollars spent for soft drink advertising rose by 28 percent, for candy and snacks by 40 percent, and for restaurants by 86 percent. The U.S. food industry is the second largest advertiser (the auto industry is number one).

U.S. Department of Agriculture figures show that the proportion of advertising money that companies spend on candy and snacks, prepared convenience foods, and soft drinks far exceeds these foods' share of the American diet. What the food industry spends just on promoting snacks and nuts matches the entire USDA's budget for nutrition research, education, and other activities.

"Twenty corporations pay for nearly three-quarters of all food advertising in the U.S.," says Ronald Cotterrill, professor of marketing at the University of Connecticut. "And they spend it to promote highly processed foods like soft drinks, cookies, and convenience foods."

THE FATTENING OF AMERICA

It's true for men and women, children and adults, whites and minorities. It's true for every state and most countries of the world. We're getting fatter. More than half of American adults – 54 percent – are now overweight. The number has climbed steadily since the early 1960s, when it was 43 percent. What's more, children are following in their parents' heavier footsteps. One out of eight school-aged kids is obese, twice the fraction of two decades ago. And experts estimate that one in four is overweight.

And growing waistlines have a growing cost.

Diabetes is the disease most closely linked to overweight. Since 1990, type 2 diabetes has jumped by 33 percent nationwide. And that's just the tip of the iceberg. "Much of the impact of the upsurge in obesity may be felt some years from now, because there is a substantial delay between the onset of obesity and the subsequent development of diabetes," says Jeffrey P. Koplan, director of the Centers for Disease Control and Prevention (CDC) in Atlanta.

Roughly 800,000 Americans – some of them adolescents – are diagnosed with diabetes each year. Among the disease's consequences: an increased risk of heart disease, stroke, blindness, high blood pressure, kidney disease, and amputations. "American lifestyles, including inactivity and poor nutrition, are having a dramatic influence on our health," says Koplan. And there's no reason to think that the obesity epidemic has hit its peak.

"Our diet is deteriorating and physical activity is declining," says Yale University obesity expert Kelly Brownell. "Our environment conspires to make both worse and worse."

What Brownell has dubbed the "toxic food environment" includes almost every gas station, shopping mall, convenience store, vending machine, ballpark, movie theater, and restaurant, all tempting people with too much of the wrong foods. Before infants are even out of their diapers, they're assaulted by TV commercials, jingles, toys, and celebrity endorsements, a whole culture, badgering them to eat junk.

"The promotion of high-fat and high-calorie foods goes on unabated," says Brownell. "Food is more accessible and cheaper than ever. I've seen two Big Macs for two dollars, that's a lot of calories for not much money." At the same time, we expend fewer calories than we used to. "We can expect more and more energy-saving devices," he adds. "Computers will become more a part of our everyday life and work. And kids are getting less physical activity because of TV, computers, and video games."

What can stem the rising tide of plus sizes? "The first step is to recognize that what we've been doing has failed," says Brownell. "We can't just blame individuals and treat them with drugs. Offering treatment to people one at a time is necessary, but for every person we remove from the obese population, a thousand people may enter it." And it's not just a matter of educating people about the dangers of obesity, Brownell notes. "There's already tremendous pressure on people to be thin, to exercise more and eat better. We can't count on people to all of a sudden change their behavior."

Instead, says Brownell, we need public policies that alter the landscape. "We could subsidize the cost of fruits and vegetables and, if necessary, tax unhealthy foods," he suggests. "We could make physical activity more accessible by opening bike paths and recreation centers."

And at the very least, we should clean up our kids' environment. "Why not balance junk-food ads aimed at kids with pro-nutrition messages?" says Brownell. "We could prohibit soft drinks and fast food from schools, and completely restructure the school-lunch program."

Brownell draws a parallel between food and cigarettes. "We used to think that smoking was just a matter of will power," he says. "Now we recognize that the tobacco industry is a powerful force that encourages people, especially young people, to smoke." Until the public sees the food industry as a comparable force, we can expect obesity rates to continue to climb.

Note: Reproduced with the permission of: Center for Science in the Public Interest. "Food Marketing Madness" and "The Fattening of America" are excerpts from an article on the Top Ten Mega-trends of 2001, as discussed by the Nutrition Action HealthLetter. You will notice that these trends are still major issues today.

Liebman, B., Schardt, D., & Jones, H. *(Jan 2001)*. Diet & Health: Ten Megatrends. Nutrition Action, 28, 3-4, 12. *(excerpts)*

Vitamins, Minerals and Water

Vitamins and Minerals

Vitamins and minerals are certainly necessary to life. In fact, "vita" is a Latin word meaning "life". Vitamins and minerals are essential nutrients that your body needs in small amounts in order to work properly. They are nutrients for the human body that are contained within food substances. Vitamins control chemical reactions within the body to convert food into energy and living tissue. They help the body use the energy nutrients, maintain normal body tissue, and act as a regulator.

Minerals are needed for several body functions, including building strong bones, transmitting nerve signals, maintaining a normal heart beat, and producing necessary hormones. We should be able to get all the vitamins and minerals we need from a proper healthy diet. However, besides the fact that most of us do not eat correctly, the road from the farm to the dinner table is not well paved. If you do choose to take supplements, make sure you are informed.

A Basic Multi-Vitamin is Good Insurance

Jump in my time machine... We are heading to 2020 - a year when this vitamin supplement business should be truly settled.

We have arrived in 2020 and our first stop is a doctor's office. In order to recommend the right multi-vitamin for you, the doctor asks you to step into the Multi-Vitamin Fiber-Optic Laser Inter-Dermal Cellular Scanner, which precisely detects all vitamin and mineral deficiencies that you might have. You will then go to a pharmacist who will concoct – with the help of a super computer, of course – a personal vitamin supplement designed specifically for your needs.

This vitamin machine was developed because researchers specializing in the roles of trace minerals in metabolism function discovered a dangerous trend as far back as the early 1990's. People were taking enormous quantities of all kinds of mineral combinations, yet no one knew for sure how much a particular person needed. Finally, the Food and Drug Administration *(FDA)* stepped in and declared, "Vitamins and minerals are like drugs, they need to be regulated and not abused." Physicians agreed. However, as of yet, vitamins, minerals, and herbal supplements are still not regulated by the FDA.

By the late 1990's, nearly all medical schools required their students to take advanced courses that included specific education about vitamins and minerals. In 1975, as I was going through my graduate program, some of the faculty of the department frowned on the use of multi-vitamins. Many of my professors believed that if you ate a healthy and well-balanced diet, then you did not need to take a multi-vitamin. They taught that humans should be able to obtain all vital nutrients from food, be it fresh, frozen or even canned. Some still hold this view.

The problem with this *(aside from the fact that most of us do not even come close to our recommended 5 to 9 servings of fruits and vegetables each day)* centers on the quality of food once it actually reaches one's plate. When was the food grown? How soon was it refrigerated after harvesting? Did it travel across the state, across the country, or across the world? How much heat and light was it exposed to on the trip from the field to the distributor to your local grocery to your dinner table? How did you cook it? Was it steamed, boiled, fried or nuked? The answers to these questions greatly affect the quality and quantity of the nutrients in the food you eat. Since much of the produce we eat these days comes from far away countries, many of these factors of are out of your control.

What CAN You Do to Get More Nutrients From Food?

What IS in your control? The fact is, you do not actually have to buy all of your fruits and vegetables from "far away lands!" Find out where and when your city's local farmers' market takes place and make an attempt to do most of your produce shopping there. The fruits and vegetables grown by local farmers in season and recently picked, and therefore are usually fresher, richer in nutrients, and tastier. They are also less likely to be coated in wax or to have been grown with pesticides. Often, they are the same cost or even cheaper, and many accept food stamps. You will learn what is in season when and become motivated to try different fruits and veggies and expand your recipe selection. Going to farmers' markets also help you to get out of the "rut" of buying the same fruits and veggies every time you go to the grocery store, which causes you to quickly get bored of them.

Plus, you will be supporting your community and local farmers by cutting out the middle-men. It is quite a good feeling and an unusual concept in this day and age, to know that your whole dollar is actually going to the farmer that grew the food, as opposed to the many distributors along the way (*not to mention the massive amounts of fuel used to fly/drive/ship the food from wherever it came from to your local store*).

What else is in your control? How you cook those vegetables! For most vegetables, boiling tends to leach the vitamins and minerals out of the vegetable and into the water. If you wind up using the water that those vitamins and minerals leach into *(as in a soup)*...great! However, if you wind up pouring that water down the drain *(as most of us do)*, then you are also pouring some of those vitamins and minerals down the drain, saying "bye, bye" to half of the reason you are eating those vegetables in the first place!

The solution? Short of becoming one of the avid members of the "raw foods diet" *(this very issue is cornerstone of why it was created)*, you can choose to lightly STEAM veggies instead of boiling the "bejesus" out of them. For a few bucks, you can buy a basic metal steamer from your grocery store, stick it in the bottom of the pot, fill the pot with water just up to the height of the steamer, and steam your veggies *(be sure to check them regularly, by poking with a knife, to avoid overcooking)*. This will help you retain more of those precious vitamins and minerals that you hope to get from eating that broccoli or carrot.

So, is a multi-vitamin and mineral supplement necessary or at least beneficial? What to do? In my humble opinion - unless you have a truly specific need - take a basic multi-vitamin. It doesn't matter if it is from a pharmacy, supermarket or health food store *(but be leery of bargain brands)*. A little "nutrition insurance" can't hurt.

We Really Are a Body of Water

"Water, water everywhere" *(and plenty to drink)*, but why should we? Fetuses begin life as cells bathed in water. This water, called amniotic fluid, surrounds the baby in the uterus and helps to protect and cushion the baby against physical injury and infection. As vital as this water is in utero, a human's need for it increases after birth. About 60 percent of your body is water, and about a quart a day is lost through breathing, sweating and waste, so you need to replace it constantly.

Why is water there, and what does it do? The water in your body serves many functions. It helps remove toxins from your body, cushions your joints, regulates your body temperature, and carries oxygen and nutrients into your cells. Without adequate amounts of water in your body, not only may you end up with terrible constipation, but your blood pressure can fall to dangerously low levels, blood clots may form, and your kidney function may become impaired.

Every cell in your body needs water, and it is important to drink 6 to 8 glasses of water a day. If you burn 2,000 calories daily through normal daily movement and mild exercise, the recommended daily allowance is six to eight cups of fluid. We often do not realize that daily food intake typically provides two to four cups of water. Of course, the more you sweat, the greater your fluid needs. The overweight person needs more water than the thin one. Larger people have larger metabolic loads, and water is a key player in metabolizing fat.

Beat the Thirst

Thirst is a feeling you truly need to be aware of, because it is the most your body can do to send the message, "Drink, you fool." It is best to not wait until you are thirsty to drink water, because by the time you start to feel the thirst, your body has already begun to become dehydrated. Extreme cases of dehydration could lead to fainting, heat exhaustion, coma or death. The key to avoiding all dehydration-related problems is to get into the habit of drinking regularly. The best way to do this? Keep a cup, bottle, or glass of water with you at all times – in your car, on your desk, in front of the TV, in the kitchen, next to your bed.

Of course, drinking fluids does not mean drinking just any fluid. Red wine may lower your cholesterol, but this is not an excuse to imbibe. Sorry folks; alcohol is not a mandatory fluid. Alcohol causes increased water loss *(diuresis)* through increased urination, and so does caffeine. Thus, if you drink a lot of caffeinated beverages *(I am hoping if this is the case, it is coffee, tea, or diet soda instead of regular soda, mochas, sweet tea, etc.)*, then you must balance those out with even more water.

Believe it or not, fruit juice is not a great substitute for water either. Before you call the Florida Citrus Commission, let me explain. We need fruit in our diet, but not as a routine thirst quencher. Fruit juice is not a substitute for natural fruit, as it has fewer nutrients, less fiber, more sugar, and more calories. The calories from fruit juices are mostly from sugars and carbohydrates. If you are going to drink fruit juice, make sure that it is "100% fruit juice" and/or with "no added sugar". Start looking at the labels, and you will be shocked to see how many fruit drinks actually have very little juice in them. Even with 100% fruit juice, LIMIT YOUR INTAKE OF FRUIT JUICE TO NO MORE THAN ONE GLASS/SERVING PER DAY *(or drink even less often if you have another sweetened drink during the course of a day)*. The rest of your fruit should come in solid form.

One way to make this one glass per day go further: dilute your juice by filling 1/4 to 1/2 of the glass with juice and the rest of it with cold water *(regular or carbonated)*. The taste may seem bland at first, but you will quickly get used to it and soon, the taste of the juice alone *(undiluted)* will seem overpowering. This works especially well with cranberry, apple or grape juice. Note: Feeding fruit juice to children in bottles, especially while they fall asleep, is a big risk for dental cavities and very bad idea. The fructose *(fruit sugar)* remains on the teeth for hours and can result in decay.

Water is clearly the best routine source of fluid. If you do not like the taste of tap water, try a filter system, home water cooler, or bottled water. If you do not want to or can not spend the money to have a filter on your faucet or under your sink, buy a water pitcher/cooler with a filter in it *(such as the ones made by Brita)* that you can keep in the fridge and refill as needed. Today, bottled water floods the market with hundreds of different products. They are either plain bottled water or with additives in the form of different flavorings, nutrients, bubbles or coloring. Many are quite expensive. Water from the faucet, on the other hand, is the cheapest drink you can get! Cost is definitely not an excuse for choosing unhealthy, sweetened drinks over water. If you typically buy bottled, instead get the recommended pitcher with disposable filter and you will save money in the long run. It is also much more environmentally friendly, because you can refill and reuse water bottles without having to waste so much plastic. If you do go for the flavored water, read the ingredients list or the nutritional facts on the label to make sure the drink does not have sugar added.

So, whether it is tap, filtered or bottled water, drink more of it routinely. Your body will appreciate it. As an added bonus, water is the medium that carries fat out of the body. So drink water - for the health of it!

Just Add Food

Foods contain water. Foods with high water content can provide taste, texture and variety and additionally, contribute to your body's fluid reservoir. Almost every food supplies fluid and helps fill your need for replacement water. At the top of the list of juicy foods are fruits and vegetables. Some "dry-sounding" foods are also good fluid sources: beans and grains such as pasta actually act as sponges as they cook and become good sources of water. Here is the water content of food by percentage:

Water content of food by percentage
Citrus fruits 91
Apples 84
Bananas......................................74
Rice and pasta 66-72
Grains 66-72
Beans...................................65-75
Fish......................................60-70
Breads 32

The Hard *(and Soft)* Facts

According to Dr. Ellie Whitney's *Nutrition Concepts and Controversies (a great book)*, hard water has high concentrations of calcium and magnesium that could help prevent osteoporosis, heart disease and hypertension. You know your water is hard if it hurts coming out of the shower head *(sorry, just kidding)*. Hard water leaves a ring around the bathtub and rock-like crystals in the tea kettle. Soft water has more sodium, which may promote hypertension, but is often preferred because it dissolves metals such as cadmium and lead from pipes.

Cadmium can block the absorption of zinc, an essential nutrient that promotes healing of tissue. Lead, of course, is a toxic metal and can damage the brain, nerves, red blood cells and digestive system.

Time to "Bone Up" on Your Calcium Knowledge

Your mother told you. Your grandmother told you. Even the media tells you. "Milk, it does the body good." Why is it so good? Let's examine the major mineral ingredient in milk and other dairy products – calcium.

Calcium, the fifth-most abundant element on earth, is everywhere. It is in limestone, in driveways and in coral from the Florida Keys. It is in the pearls you wish you had around your neck and the marbles in your head. It is in your teeth *(hopefully you still have them)* and of course, in your bones.

It "does the body good" because it helps our heart to beat regularly, our blood pressure to be regulated, our blood to coagulate, our muscles to contract, our glands to secrete and our cells to divide. It helps your bones to grow, too, especially in infancy and in adolescence.

Bones Keep Growing

In adolescence, it just doesn't seem cool to drink milk. Children become more independent, peers take over and sodas enter the scene. Your child, who drank milk fairly voluntarily until age 10, now refuses. Leafy green vegetables *(which are also high in calcium)*, you can forget *(unless you are extremely lucky or your child has an affinity for Popeye)*.

The problem is that 10 years of drinking milk isn't enough. Bone mass continues to be added until about the age of 19, and density of the bones in the thigh and upper spine can start to decline as early as age 18. Children need more calcium from ages 9 to 17 than at any other time in their lives. During this growth period, children experience the greatest muscular, skeletal and reproductive development. By age 10, height increases two inches a year in girls and peaks at 2 1/4 to 2 1/2 inches a year by age 12, on average. Boys grow an average of 2 inches a year at age 12 and about 3 inches a year at age 14.

For both sexes, 37 percent of the adult skeletal mass is accumulated between the ages of 11 and 14. From age 2 through adolescence, they need approximately 800 mg of calcium daily. Most of us have observed that infants triple their weight over their first year of life. This is primarily due to bone-mass increase. Adults of both sexes need approximately 1,000 mg of calcium a day, and post-menopausal women need 1,500 mg daily.

Ok, So Now I Know That I Need Calcium, Where Do I Get It?

Obviously, diary products – particularly low-fat ones – are a good source of calcium. A cup of skim milk or a cup of yogurt contains about 300 mg of calcium. An ounce of cheese has 280 mg of calcium. In addition to milk and other dairy products, there are a variety of foods that contain calcium. These foods can help both children and adults get sufficient levels of calcium in their diet.

Leafy green vegetables like broccoli, kale and spinach are high in calcium. But two problems with these are: a) it is often hard to get children to eat these and b) they contain oxalates, which bind with the calcium and limit the body's ability to absorb it. Still, they are necessary in your diet. Other foods containing calcium that kids *(and probably you)* are more likely to eat include: oranges, peanuts, baked beans, peas, salmon, almonds and black beans.

Still, dairy products are the most absorbable form of calcium. Vitamin D, magnesium and phosphorus, all present in dairy products, help the body absorb calcium. Some other foods, such as breads and cereals are fortified with vitamin D. Natural sunlight absorbed through the skin also causes the body to synthesize vitamin D. People over 60 years old would benefit from vitamin D3 along with their calcium.

If you are lactose-intolerant, have issues with congestion/sinuses, or do not like milk, use an alternative such as soy milk or rice milk that is fortified with calcium and vitamin D *(it will say on the label)*. Many varieties of soy milk (like Silk) have just as much calcium as regular milk. My favorite is Silk's Light Vanilla.

Supplementary Knowledge

Calcium supplements are the last alternative if you cannot *(lactose intolerance or milk allergies)* or will not *(stubbornness)* consume dairy products, but they should not be solely relied upon. Today's recommendation is to take a calcium supplement with a meal.

If you do not eat dairy products, find calcium and vitamin D-fortified dairy-alternative products that you can consume daily. If you are not satisfied with the selection at your local grocery, check out a health food store near you for a wider variety and products you did not even know existed!

In the beginning, we want to grow, so we need calcium. In later years, we do not want to shrink or break bones, so we need calcium. You will be better off, just like your mother told you, if you drink your milk *(or soy milk)* and eat your veggies, dahling!

Holiday Eating

(More creative titles for this chapter include: "When Carols Give Rise to Perils" or "Egg Nog, Pumpkin Pie, Fatty Thigh" or the Jewish version: "Fried Latkes, Gelt, and Guilt")

Let's start with the "eatingest" time of the entire year: Thanksgiving through Christmas, with a little New Year's Eve celebration thrown in. When Thanksgiving stares us in the face and Hanukkah, Christmas and Kwanza are soon to follow, the holiday eating frenzy begins.

But there is no need to get crazy here. You do not have to accept the many extra pounds that Santa will gladly bring you and that much of the population simply gives into. Control and a little planning are keys for you to get a handle on your love handles.

Thanksgiving: The Truly American Holiday

Thanksgiving, the first major feast of the "holiday eating season," does not have to be a Thursday through Sunday food marathon. Turkey Day can consist of just one major splurge meal, but most of us turn it into more.

One big suggestion is to eat at midday, leaving some daylight to go for a walk afterward. A walk within an hour and a half of the meal will help speed up your metabolism, so it can digest the massive amount of food. So if you take a walk for 30 minutes within one to one and a half hours after that large meal, your metabolism will speed up to compensate for the volumes you just enjoyed and hopefully, result in no weight gain.

Thanksgiving is supposed to be just one meal, on one day, although many of us "give thanks" for three or four days, depending on how far we have traveled and how long we have been away from "momma's cookin'!" Have a plan of attack for just that meal. For most, the Turkey Day meal is between 12 to 2 p.m. or 4 to 6 p.m. It is never for breakfast, and it is usually not on time. So the first suggestion is to definitely eat breakfast earlier that day *(no, do not skip it in attempt to eat less)*. Also, go for a walk, if you can, before breakfast. Both of these strategies will help get your metabolism get going before you even sit down for your overindulgence.

If the meal is at 1 or 2 p.m. and you normally eat lunch around 12 p.m., have a light starch-based snack. A piece of toast with jam or light peanut butter one hour before the meal will take the edge off. Finally, accept the fact that the Thanksgiving meal is normally an out of control feeding frenzy and enjoy it. Try limiting your serving size by using just one large soup spoon for each dish that you want to partake in. By doing this, you can eat some of everything you want, just not too much of it. Be sure to go for something green as well, such as a salad, greens, or green beans. Seconds? Go for the one item that you want the most.

Dessert: Ah, yes, pumpkin, apple, pecan, and sweet potato pie... Go for a very small piece *(sliver)* of each of the various pies that you want to try. This way, you can get variety and the tastes you want, but not keep going back for "just one more." Keep in mind: You should be able to fit all small pieces on the same dessert plate. After the meal, put all the food out of sight and leave the kitchen, so it is not constantly calling your name.

The above suggestions can also be applied to Christmas Day and other major holidays.

Ah, Those Holiday Parties

So now you have made it to December, only to hear an Olympian voice in your head cry out, "Let the *(food)* games begin!" At 7 p.m., you enter the cocktail party and nonchalantly saunter over to the hors d'oeuvres table. It is early evening after work and you have not yet eaten dinner, so your stomach is growling. Picking up a petite plate, you gather a variety of goodies. Traveling along the table, you quickly load your plate so it looks like a volcano about to erupt with taste treats.

You hit it off with someone and begin chatting *(with the eating following right behind because it subdues your nervousness)*. But you are standing and eating and you forgot all about Nutrition Rule #444 1/2: NEVER STAND AND EAT. It is neither comfortable nor satisfying to eat standing up, with more food and drink a mere arm's length away, and you will probably finish your plate before you even realize that you started eating. Instead, go sit down with your friend. And before you start piling on the goodies off the table, "scout out" the food first to find out what is there. This way, you can selectively indulge. To truly prevent a full dinner of desserts and high-fat finger food, have a light, fast meal, such as a baked potato, before you get to the party. This takes the edge off and can help prevent a potential binge.

Alcoholic beverages can cause problems year-round, but the dangers seem even more prevalent during the holidays. Try choosing either an alcoholic beverage or a dessert, but not both. Drink in moderation, if you drink at all, and please don't drink and drive.

Holiday Baking and Healthy Alternatives

Holiday baking is certainly a pleasure for both the baker and the "bakee." But the best-laid baking plans often go astray because of the "one for them, one for me" sorting method. One suggestion is to not bake at all *(I know, no fun)*. Another option is to eat a reasonable meal before you bake, then package the goodies and send them off to their lucky recipients to get them out of sight *(it sounds bad, but if you are really having a hard time not keeping some of those cookies you just made for your friends, just picture them having gained 10 pounds come January 1st and you having gained none!)* Following are some suggestions for healthy holiday snacks.

Healthy Holiday Snacks

1. CHESTNUTS *(roasted)*
   Chestnuts are a low-fat, low-calorie nut, high in fiber, cholesterol-free and nutritionally similar to brown rice. Cook at 425 degrees for 20-25 minutes. Remember to use the knife to cut an X on the top side of the shell to prevent nut from exploding.

2. LOWER CALORIE EGGNOG
   Substitute with low-fat, fat-free, skim or soy milk or dilute with water. Silk actually now produces a non-dairy egg nog for the holiday season. Sprinkling nutmeg on top of any lower-fat version really will help it to taste more like the real thing!

3. CRANBERRIES *(sauce, relish salsa, sherbet)*
   Cranberries can help lower LDL *(bad cholesterol)* and have antioxidants that help prevent urinary infections, kidney

stones, heart disease and cancer. However, most store-bought dried cranberries have added sugar, so do not overdo it. For a quick snack:, mix 1/2 cup "craisins" and 4 cups light microwave popcorn.

4. CHRISTMAS PEARS and HOLIDAY CLEMENTINES *(small mandarins)* Pears are rich in soluble fiber and act as body detoxifier. Pears are low on the glycemic index and high in vitamins A and C and Phosphorous. Clementines are loaded with vitamin C, folic acid and fiber.

5. LOW-FAT LATKES *(potato pancakes that are a traditional food of Hanukkah)*

   Use Yukon potatoes *(for a buttery flavor)*, substitute eggs with egg whites, use olive oil, and bake instead of fry. As a topping, use low-fat or fat-free sour cream instead of regular sour cream or use the other popular latke topping...applesauce!

6. BITE-SIZED KASHI BARS

   Cut Kashi Bars into bite sized pieces and lightly sprinkle with powered sugar. The Trail mix Kashi Bars are 140 calories in a bar. They contain 7 whole grains, almonds and cranberries and no trans fat.

7. PUMPKIN *(puree, pie, soup)*

   It is a vegetable and it is also delicious. Pumpkin is loaded with vitamins A, C, K and E. It also is rich in alpha and beta-carotene, potassium and zinc. When making a pie, use low-fat milk and whole wheat flour in the crust.

8. TRAIL MIX *(Light version)*

   Mix, in equal portions: Honeynut Cheerios, raisins, popcorn, and small rice cakes *(broken up)*. Cheerios are toasted whole grain oats that have been proven to lower blood cholesterol and are a source of heart healthy soluble fiber.

9. DARK CHOCOLATE COVERED STRAWBERRIES *(but beware of calories!!)*

Dark chocolate is medically proven to lower blood pressure *(from plant phenols)*, and it contains antioxidants. No similar benefit from milk or white chocolate. Dip a few strawberries in dark melted chocolate.

10. ANGELFOOD CAKE

It is fat-free and low in calories. The light and airy cake can be gussied up with a simple garnish of fresh fruit.

The Office: Why Do Co-Workers Bring SO Many Treats to Work?

You have steered clear of over-indulging at parties and at home, but there is one other major hurdle to jump, the office food spread. And it is hard, because you work there, for Pete's sake! If you work at a doctor's office, a government office, or a large corporate office, many people experience the "Twelve Days of Christmas" at work, also known as, "Let's see who can gain the most weight before Christmas." My advice is to encourage your co-workers not to indulge in that custom or to alter it to have a healthier theme every day but Friday. Bring it up at an office meeting.

Instead of co-workers bringing in cookies, suggest the idea of "Soup Day," in which a few people bring in a different hearty soup. Or have a "pot luck day." Make a sign-up sheet denoting who brings a meat dish, who brings a starch, and which two bring in vegetable plates *(the rest of the co-workers can sign up the next time around)*. It is more satisfying to be treated to an actual meal, rather than just a dessert, isn't it? Plus, I am SURE that you are not the only one in the office who is trying to lose weight. Try a "Healthy Snack Day" or a low-fat themed day. You could all find and try new things that actually taste good to eat but are healthy. An additional suggestion is to just have some hard candy around the office – candy canes and peppermint balls are good choices. Of course, you can see why I am not invited to drop by everyone's offices prior to Christmas! The healthy holiday snacks previously listed are also good choices to bring into the office. Share your healthy knowledge!

Food crops up everywhere in the office, and it is very difficult to ignore. Your intentions may be honorable, but major willpower is being tested here. Sometimes you feel like you are doing well in skipping the fudge on one desk, even if you have two cookies off the next. Suggest that the holiday treats in your office be kept in one place and not scattered everywhere. This way, people who want to stay in control at least have a fighting chance. And if all willpower fades, compensate another way. Find a partner and take a lunchtime walk throughout the holidays. This will minimize the damage and may get you started on a healthy habit.

Another crazy idea is to create a healthy little competition for your workplace: bring in or purchase an office pre-holiday scale. Place it in the privacy of the "Snack Room." The person who gains the least amount of weight during the holidays gets $10 from every other fellow employee!

The holidays should be fun and healthy but also include some indulgences *(I'm not Scrooge McNutritionist)*. So enjoy the holidays, but remember that the average weight gain from Thanksgiving to New Year's Day is 5 to 7 pounds! HOWEVER, THIS DOES NOT HAVE TO HAPPEN TO YOU! Eat, drink, walk and be wary!

Leftovers

If you did the cooking, send home all the leftovers *(which normally would be calling your name)* with your guests or family. Get all those high-calorie items such as desserts, stuffing, brown-sugar laden sweet potatoes, and the dark meat of the turkey (the fattest part) out of the house. Another way to handle leftovers is do not have any in the first place. Go out to a favorite local restaurant for the Thanksgiving meal. Yea! Smart, and no hassles. No dishes either...hmm...

You Say You Want a (Weight) Revolution (Well, we all want to change our weights...)

(The above is yet another allusion to classic songs of the 60's...in case you are from a different era or simply don't get my strange humor.)

Finally, holiday parties are coming to a close and office binges are winding down. Santa has delivered his loot and your initially mild weight-related guilt is growing out of control. Get that right hand up and repeat after me, "I will tell the truth, the whole truth and nothing but the truth, so help me lard." Are you ready for your New Year's Revolution *(or is it resolution)*?

The New Year's Revolution can also be known as the Revolving Diet Syndrome *(RDS)*. People look to RDS to arrest the major guilt associated with the five-week feeding frenzy from Thanksgiving Day through New Year's. Losing weight is a major undertaking, but with the right attitude, this year CAN be your year to succeed. Seriously folks, binge dieting may work for a while, but by surrendering to it, you are doomed to ultimate failure. The "gain, loose, gain" cycle is not fun, in fact, it is very frustrating and self-defeating.

For a Resolution to Work, It Must be Accompanied by a Plan

The best way to stay with your resolution is to take one habit or behavior at a time and work on it and only it. For example, let's say you eat too quickly *(and because of that you eat too much)*. By eating more slowly, your stomach has enough time to let your brain know that you have had enough. You can be satisfied with less food, and you may be surprised at how good your meals taste when you actually eat slowly instead of inhaling.

So here is the technique: If you can, use your opposite hand to eat for two weeks. *(You can wear a bib and feel free to skip this in restaurants if you're not steady!)* Go back to your usual hand after 14 days, but keep up your slower pace. And make sure your "gun isn't loaded" *(i.e. don't load up your fork with the next bite while you are still chewing the previous one).*

Ok, now you are eating slower. Mission completed. Good job. Next habit to change is not snacking as soon as you get in the door from work. Many of us enter the house through the kitchen and head straight to the refrigerator, to "make sure everything is still there." Well, it was, until the snacking started. Go into the bedroom, bathroom or living room instead, as soon as you get home, to break that habit. Pet the dog, change your clothes, wash up or read the mail, just please don't go into the kitchen. And if any of you keep a stash of food next to your bed, or in your purse or briefcase, don't go there either!

There Are Many Bad Habits We Can Break

Are you standing up and eating? Eating the wrong food and a lot of it? Skipping exercising? Rewarding yourself with food or rewarding others' behavior with food? Do you eat when you are depressed, angry or frustrated? Do you skip breakfast? Do you frequent fast food places? Do you have no routine with when and how much you eat? Do you graze in the kitchen?

Personalize this plan to your needs: Write down the five habits you recognize as the biggest problems. Then, set up your plan of attack and your time frame for doing it, and get going. Gradual change will help you create new, healthy habits. It is human nature to look for a quick fix. When it comes to losing weight and keeping it off, there are no shortcuts. Be wary of weight loss promises that sound too good to be true...they probably are. Short-term diets never work. So plan on losing weight slowly and realize you must change your habits and behaviors that caused you to gain the weight in the first place. You must develop new habits that you will be able to maintain for the rest of your life.

Good luck and have a happy, healthy New Year!

Fiber Freddy "Sez":

Fiber has been on my mind since at least 1975, when the Leon County Food Co-Op produced a newsletter which carried my column, "Fiber Freddy Sez." *(Cheesy title? Yes. Informative? Quite.)* However, I am surprised that three decades later, I am still witnessing well-educated, exercise-conscious people eating sandwiches on white bread. Yet choosing whole wheat bread over white bread is one of the simplest, most effective small changes you can make in the process of eating a healthier diet.

What Does "Whole Grain" Mean?

All grains start out as whole grains, made up of three parts: the bran, the endosperm, and the germ. The bran *(protective outer shell)* contains B-vitamins and most of the fiber; the endosperm contains starch, protein, and some vitamins and minerals; the germ *(seed)* contains B vitamins, vitamin E, some protein, minerals, healthy oils and antioxidants. Through milling and processing, the outer *(nutrient-rich)* layers are often discarded. Enriched "white" flour is more processed than whole wheat flour, and by the time the "white" flour is done being processed, it contains only the endosperm. Thus, it is missing the majority of the fiber, B vitamins, extra protein, and some of the healthy minerals and oils. For health benefits, we want the "whole" kernel, not just the inside. If bread producers left the grain alone, they would not need to "enrich" it. The germ itself is rich in vitamins and minerals.

How Can I Tell if a Food is "Whole Grain"?

Think brown! But be careful when using the "color rule" for bread. Just because bread is brown does not always mean it is whole-grain. It is a good clue, but bread may be brown for other reasons, such as being made with molasses or caramel food coloring! Choosing the right bread may be even more confusing because of misleading or confusing labeling. The package might read "made with whole wheat" but actually have only a percentage of whole wheat flour in it.

The Whole Grain Council has now created two official stamps to make it easier to find real whole wheat products. The Council's "Whole Grain Stamp" tells you that the majority of the product is made with whole grains. Still, the best way to be sure that what you are getting has the highest fiber content, look for the "100% Whole Grain" claim on the package. With bread, for instance, I recommend only buying bread that is 100% whole wheat (*whole wheat is one type of whole grain*).

If you do not see "100% whole wheat," another way to tell is by looking at the ingredients list. If the words "WHOLE WHEAT" or another type of grain with the word "WHOLE" before it (*such as whole rye or whole oats*) are not part of the FIRST ingredient listed, then it is not a 100% whole-grain food. If "whole wheat" is listed as the second ingredient, then you have no idea whether it makes up 5% or 45% of the food product. A product that says "multigrain" is also unclear as to how much of it is actually whole grain. You need to look at the ingredients list.

If the first ingredient is any of the following, then it is probably whole grain: whole wheat, whole grain wheat, whole grain barley, whole grain corn (*or whole cornmeal*), whole grain buckwheat, whole grain rye, OR oatmeal, wheat berries, cracked wheat, whole oats, brown rice, wild rice, bulgur, or popcorn.

It is easy to be fooled, but now you know what to look for!

There really is a big difference in fiber content. Whole wheat bread is typically 5.1 percent fiber, while white bread is only 2.7 percent fiber.

Why is Fiber Important?

Dietary fiber is the material that remains after plant foods pass through the intestinal tract. Fiber has important benefits for health, particularly through its effect on the digestive system. There are numerous diseases directly related to a deficiency of fiber in the diet. These diseases/disorders are common ones, such as high blood pressure, bowel disorders, hemorrhoids, varicose veins, appendicitis, diverticulitis, colitis, stroke and cancer of the colon. It also decreases heart disease by decreasing cholesterol and may decrease the amount of insulin needed by diabetics. Because it makes you feel fuller, it also helps you lose weight by not eating as much.

Soluble VS. Insoluble Fiber and Their Effects on Digestion

Not all fiber is the same, and fiber comes in two forms: soluble and insoluble. All plant materials contain both types of fiber, but some sources contain more of one than the other. In general, if a plant food seems rough, stringy, has a tough skin, hull, peel, pod or seed, it is likely high in insoluble fiber. For fruits, vegetables and legumes, peeling, chopping, cooking and pureeing them will significantly minimize the impact of their insoluble fiber. Both soluble and insoluble fiber are undigested. They are, therefore, not absorbed into the bloodstream. Instead of being used for energy, fiber is excreted from our bodies. Soluble fiber forms a gel when mixed with liquid, while insoluble fiber does not. Insoluble fiber passes through our intestines largely intact. Eating a variety of foods rich in fiber every day will ensure you get adequate levels of both soluble and insoluble fiber.

Insoluble fiber is important in keeping people "regular" and prevents constipation. It also speeds up toxic waste removal through the colon and helps prevent colon cancer. Insoluble fiber *(unable to be dissolved in water)* is especially important in weight loss because it helps satisfy the appetite. It helps satisfy the appetite because it takes longer to chew, allowing your body more time to register that it is no longer hungry; it also feels like a larger quantity but has lower calories. Insoluble fiber promotes regularity by adding bulk to your stool and softening it. Fiber helps create a soft stool that causes less pressure on the muscles of the intestines *(not a recommended subject for discussion at dinner!)* Fiber from grains also hastens the speed in which food and bacteria travel through the intestines, preventing bacteria from growing and forming polyps in the intestines. Sources for insoluble fiber include: green leafy vegetables, fruit skins and root vegetable skins, corn, seeds, and nuts, but whole grains are the best and most convenient option for increasing regularity.

Soluble fiber reduces levels of cholesterol in the blood *(thus reducing the risk of heart disease)* and also reduces the rate at which glucose enters the bloodstream *(e.g. helps regulate blood sugar)*. Because these fibers bind with fatty acids, they sit in your stomach and allow the sugar to be broken down. Soluble fiber is abundant in dried beans and peas, lentils, barley, oats/oat bran, flax seed, nuts, and in many fruits (such as apples and oranges) and vegetables *(such as carrots)*.

In addition to fiber, water and exercise also help improve bowel movements. You should focus on drinking 6-8 glasses of water a day. Fiber alone isn't enough. You must drink enough fluid to help the fiber do its job *(fiber is often measured by its water holding capacity)*. You could do a good job at getting plenty of fiber but still be constipated from not having enough water in your system.

How Much Fiber and Whole Grains Should I Eat?

The United States Department of Agriculture considers adequate daily fiber intake for children ages 4 to 8 years old to be 25 grams. For males who are 14 to 50 years old, 38 grams is considered adequate intake. For males 50+ years of age, adequate daily intake is 30 grams of fiber. For females who are 9 to 50 years old, adequate daily intake of fiber is between 25 to 26 grams *(slightly higher during pregnancy or lactation)*. For females who are 50+ years of age, adequate intake is 21 grams.[24]

The USDA's 2005 Dietary Guidelines came up with an easy recommendation slogan: "MAKE HALF YOUR GRAINS WHOLE." This suggests that at least half of all the grains you eat should be whole grains *(instead of "enriched" grains or products made with "white" flour)*. Specific recommendations differ slightly based on gender and age, but women between 31 and 50 years old should eat 6 servings of grains per day *(at least 3 of those should be whole grains)* and men of the same age should eat about 7 servings of grains per day *(at least 3.5 of those should be whole grains)*. The recommendations are similar for women and men who are younger *(14 to 30 years old)* or older *(51+ years)*. Yet, the average American eats less than one serving daily of whole grains, and over 40% of Americans do not eat whole grains at all![25]

Focus on eating at least 3 servings of whole grains per day. The more you can substitute whole-grain products for other grains, the better. A slice of bread, a cup of whole grain cereal, or 1/2 cup of brown rice or whole wheat pasta are examples of one serving of whole grains. In trying to eat 3 servings per day, a good guideline is to try to have one serving per meal. At breakfast, try: whole grain cereal, oatmeal, whole wheat toast or English muffin, or whole grain pancakes or waffles. At lunch, try: a sandwich or wrap on whole wheat bread, pita, or tortilla. At dinner, try including: whole-grain pasta, whole-grain bread, brown or wild rice, bulgur, or barley.

How Can I Eat More Fiber?

What do the peel of an apple, the skin of a potato, lettuce, broccoli, whole wheat bread, dried beans, brown rice, and most vegetables and most fruits have in common? Give up? FIBER! Those little cells that make celery so stiff.

Here are some suggestions for increasing fiber in your diet:

- Increase your vegetable portions at meals. You will get more nutrients, less calories and feel fuller.
- Try to eat fruit at every meal; canned is fine, but get the kind that is packed in juice *(or "no sugar added")* instead of syrup.
- Do not peel apples, peaches, pears or potatoes!
- Eat a whole orange, instead of just drinking the juice.
- Add fruit and nuts to muffins, pancakes and breads.
- Add berries, nuts, chickpeas, artichokes or beans to salads.
- Eat high fiber, whole-grain cereal *(or oatmeal)* on most mornings. Look at the labels and compare grams of fiber in the store before buying. Add fruit and nuts.
- Eat 100% whole-grain breads. Check the labels and the ingredients list to be sure they are really 100% whole-grain.
- Cook vegetables only until tender *(still crisp)* or eat raw.

- Buy whole-grain products such as whole wheat pastas, bagels, muffins, pancakes/waffles, pitas, and even burrito wraps.
- Use whole grains in your cooking; choose brown rice, wild rice, or barley instead of white rice.
- Exchange beans for ground meat in recipes for tacos or chili and tofu crumbles for ground meat in recipes for spaghetti sauce or lasagna.
- Eat high fiber snacks such as: fruit, raw vegetables, nuts, whole-grain granola bars, whole-grain crackers, whole-grain pretzels, and light popcorn *(yes, popcorn is a whole grain!)*.

Dietary Values of Fiber in Food
(Percentage by weight per 100 grams)

Cereals %		Leaf Vegetables	%
Wheat bran	44.0	Spinach	6.3
Wholemeal flour	9.6	Broccoli	2.9
Brown flour	7.5	Greens	3.8
white flour	3.0	Brussel sprouts	2.9
Soya flour	14.3	Cabbage	1.8
Sweetcorn (canned)	5.7	Cauliflower	1.8
Corn-on-the-cob	4.7	Celery	1.8
White rice	0.8	Lettucel	.5
Brown rice	5.5		
		Root Vegetables	**%**
Bread	**%**	Carrots	3.0
Wholemeal	8.5	Beet roots	2.5
Brown	5.1	Potatoes, baked in skins	2.5
White	2.7	Potatoes, boiled	2.0
Breakfast Cereals	**%**	**Legumes**	**%**
All Bran	26.7	Peas, frozen, boiled	12.0
Puffed Wheat	15.4	Beans, boiled	7.4
Weetabix	12.7	Peas, canned	6.3
Shredded Wheat	12.3	Broad beans	5.1
Cornflakes	11.0	Lentils	3.7
Muesli	7.4	Runner beans	3.4
Grapenuts	7.0		
Sugar Puffs	6.1	**Fruits**	**%**
Special K	5.5	Dates, dried	8.7
Rice Krispies	4.5	Blackberries	7.3
Porridge	0.8	Raisins	6.8
		Cranberries	4.2
Biscuits	**%**	Bananas	3.4
Crispbread rye	11.7	Pears, fresh	3.3
		Strawberries	2.2
Nuts	**%**	Plums	2.1
Almonds	14.3	Apples	2.0
Coconut, fresh	13.6	Oranges	2.0
Peanuts	8.1	Tomatoes, raw	1.5
Hazel nuts	6.1	Pineapple	1.2
		Grapefruit	0.6

SOURCE:*Eat Right - To Stay Healthy and Enjoy Life More* by
Denis Burkitt, M.D., 1979, Arco Pub. Co.

Know Your Cholesterol
What is Cholesterol?

Cholesterol is a fatty substance that is produced by the liver. It is also found in foods that we eat that are high in saturated fat. Fatty meats, egg yolks, shellfish, and whole milk dairy products are all high in saturated fats. So cholesterol comes from two sources: (a) your body *(partially influenced by genetics)* and (b) the food that you eat. *(In other words, you can blame either your uncle Harold OR the burger and fries you grabbed on the way home).*

Cholesterol is not all bad. Our bodies need some cholesterol to function. It is a vital part of the structure and functioning of our cells, and it is needed in the formation of certain hormones. But too much cholesterol in the blood may increase your risk of coronary heart disease, which leads to a heart attack or stroke. Cholesterol that sticks to the walls of your arteries is called plaque. Plaque on your artery walls narrows or blocks your arteries, making it harder *(or even impossible)* for the blood to get through.

Cholesterol travels through the bloodstream packaged inside a protein called lipoprotein. Two important kinds of lipoprotein are low density lipoprotein *(LDL)* and high density lipoprotein *(HDL)*. LDL cholesterol is commonly called "bad cholesterol" because it is associated with increased risk of heart attack by depositing cholesterol on the artery wall. HDL cholesterol, commonly called "good cholesterol," extracts cholesterol from the artery walls and disposes them through the liver.

Cholesterol and Food

In order to lower the cholesterol in our diet, we should reduce our caloric intake and also eat fewer fats from animal sources and more from nuts or vegetable oils, especially olive oil. Olive oil protects us from heart disease with its high content of antioxidant substances. We should eat more of the soluble fiber found in fruits and vegetables, beans, peas and oats, and try to incorporate fish into our diet at least once or twice a week.

An Aside on Fish: Benefits & Concerns

There has been much concern and confusion recently regarding the benefits of and potential concerns about eating fish. Fish is a great source of low-fat protein, and some fish contain significant amounts of the heart-healthy omega-3 oil. Omega-3 is a fatty acid that thins your blood, therefore lessening your chance for clogged arteries. By educating yourself on which and how much fish to eat, you can gain the important benefits from fish and worry less about the potential hazards. It is recommended to eat fish at least twice a week. Fish that contain the highest levels of omega-3 are: salmon, tuna, halibut, herring, sardines, mackerel, and trout *(and for shellfish: mussels and oysters)*.

The Environmental Protection Agency *(EPA)* says that the risk from mercury by eating fish and shellfish is not a health concern for most people. Women who are pregnant, women who might become pregnant, nursing mothers and young children are still encouraged to eat fish once or twice per week *(it is important for children's development)* but to be slightly more careful. The EPA's recommendations for these high-risk groups are to: (a) not eat shark, swordfish, king mackerel, or tilefish because they contain the highest amounts of mercury, (b) eat up to 12 ounces *(2 average meals)* a week of a variety of fish and shellfish that are low in mercury *(such as canned "light" tuna, salmon, shrimp, pollock, and catfish)* and (c) check local advisories regarding fish that are caught locally by friends or family members (*and if no advisory is available, do not eat locally-caught fish more than once per week*). Tuna steak and canned albacore (*"white"*) tuna have higher mercury levels than canned "light" tuna.[27]

In summary, make an attempt to include fish in your diet twice a week. It is much lower in saturated fats than other meats and has important omega-3 oils. Be aware of which fish contain the highest levels of mercury and only eat those fish occasionally. Smaller fish have fewer contaminants, due to their shorter life spans and how they eat in the ocean. Pregnant or nursing women, or women who may become pregnant, should follow the EPA's guidelines (*above*) but should still include fish in their diets because it is important for neonatal development.

Cholesterol-Lowering Medication

There are five types of cholesterol-lowering medications. They all work in different ways. Simply put, these are the ways:

1) By causing your body to make less cholesterol
2) By slowing the liver's production of chemicals that make LDL (*"bad" cholesterol*)
3) By breaking down particles that make triglycerides
4) By reducing the amount of cholesterol from the foods that you eat
5) By binding bile in the body and using more cholesterol

Unfortunately, each type of cholesterol-lowering medication (*like every medication*) has its own side effects. Some of these side effects may include: muscle weakness and heart failure, cramps, stiffness, increased risk of nerve damage, headache, hives, increased heartbeat, itching, swelling of eyelids, face or lips, low back pain or side pain, hoarseness, possible increased risk of breast cancer, difficult urination, nausea, possible link to memory loss, and sunlight sensitivity *(this is not a complete list and as with any medication, you should discuss with your physician which options may be best for you).*

Because of the potential side effects associated with cholesterol-lowering drugs, most health authorities recommend that dietary modification *(changing your diet)* be attempted first. Sometimes your health care provider will give you 3 to 6 months to lower your body's cholesterol production and then re-test and determine, in consideration of your other risk factors *(personal medical history, family medical history, etc.),* whether medications are necessary.

Everyone needs to manage their cholesterol. It is, however, even more important for some groups of individuals, including:

1. People who smoke
2. Males over 45
3. Females over 55
4. People with diabetes
5. People with high blood pressure
6. People with a personal or family history of heart disease

Even if you are prescribed medication to lower your cholesterol, you should do the following:

1. Follow a cholesterol-lowering diet
2. Lose weight
3. Increase your activity, exercise
4. Stop smoking

These lifestyle changes could lessen the amount of medication needed or make the medicine you are taking work better. Some people can actually lower their cholesterol levels through lifestyle changes alone, to the point where medication is not even needed.

Heart Disease Risk Predictors

Today, most physicians will request a yearly Lipid Profile *(through drawing and testing blood)* to determine your risk of coronary heart disease. Your cholesterol levels change with time, and it is usually difficult to tell, solely based on symptoms, whether or not your levels are high. The Lipid Profile includes measurements of total cholesterol, HDL-cholesterol *(often called the "good" cholesterol)*, LDL-cholesterol *(often called the "bad" cholesterol)* and triglycerides. If you have not had your cholesterol tested recently, you should discuss with your health care provider about having this test done.

In addition to the Lipid Profile, there are additional and possibly more accurate tests to help determine if you need medications. An article in *Environmental Nutrition* (August, 2002) titled "Leaving cholesterol in the dust: New ways to prevent heart disease" focused on the fact that half of all heart attacks occur in people with normal cholesterol and that there is much attention and debate concerning whether or not other diagnostic blood markers should be regularly checked among healthy individuals for the purpose of monitoring or helping prevent the risk of heart disease.[28] Some of these other diagnostic methods that are up for discussion include blood tests monitoring levels of homocysteine and C-reactive protein. A summary of the article's discussion on these two blood markers follows:

Homocysteine: Although high levels of the amino acid homocysteine have long been linked to heart disease, there are no studies yet that show lowering it can make a difference. There is also speculation that elevated blood homocysteine may be the result of, as opposed to a cause of, arteriosclerosis. Most experts still recommend keeping homocysteine levels low by increasing your intake of vitamins B6, B12, and especially folate, through eating dark leafy greens, lentils, dried beans and orange juice *(for* *folate)*, eating bananas, whole grains, nuts and seeds *(for vitamin B6)*, eating low-fat dairy and fortified cereals *(for vitamin B12)*, and limiting animal protein, as well as taking a multi-vitamin.[28]

C-Reactive Protein: The article discusses a high-sensitivity test, called a CRP test, that can determine if one has high levels of C-Reactive Protein *(CRP)*. High levels, which can occur even if a person's cholesterol is normal or low, can indicate the presence of inflammation in the arteries and that built-up plaque is vulnerable to rupture, which could cause a heart attack. Like with homocysteine, although there is no direct evidence that lowering CRP reduces risk of heart disease, attempts to lower it can't hurt. Besides medication, other recommended methods of reducing CRP levels included: exercising 30 to 60 minutes daily, eating a healthy diet, losing weight if you are overweight, eating less protein and drinking less alcohol, and eating foods with anti-inflammatory benefits, such as salmon, light tuna, flaxseed oil, and olive oil.[28]

EN's Guide to Heart Disease Risk Predictors		
(Presented roughly in order of their probable availability in an ordinary lab.)		

Blood Component	What Test Reveals	How to Reduce Risk
LDL-Cholesterol	A high level signals too many carriers transporting cholesterol to artery walls.	Limit saturated and trans fats by limiting full-fat dairy products, red meats, poultry skin, stick margarine, cookies, crackers and fast-food French fries.
HDL-Cholesterol	A low level indicates too few carriers transporting cholesterol away from artery walls.	Exercise regularly. Alcoholic drinks may be beneficial, but keep to one/day (women), two/day (men).

Triglycerides	A high level may mean smaller, denser LDL's, fewer HDL's and sluggish blood flow.	Limit saturated and trans fats (see above); replace with monounsaturated fats, like olive and canola oils and nuts. Cut back on refined carbohydrates, like sweets, soft drinks and white bread. Limit alcoholic drinks to one/day (women), two/day (men). Maintain a healthy weight and exercise regularly.
Homocysteine	A high level means a lot of artery-clogging plaque is present.	Eat dark leafy greens, dried beans, orange juice, asparagus and spinach for folate. Eat bananas, whole grains, nuts and seeds for vitamin B6. Eat low-fat dairy and fortified cereals for vitamin B12. Take a multi for all three B vitamins. Limit meat to limit intake of methionine.

243

C-Reactive Protein		A high level on the high-sensitivity form of test signals blood vessel inflammation and greater likelihood of rupture.		Eat salmon, mackerel, albacore tuna, sardines, walnuts and flaxseed for omega-3 fats. Maintain a healthy weight and exercise regularly. Limit alcoholic drinks to one/day (women), two/day (men). Don't follow high-protein diets.
Lipoprotein(a)		The higher the number, the more LDL's and potential for blood clots.		Discuss medication options with doctor.
Small, Dense LDL's		The smaller, denser LDL's, the more harmful free radicals created.		(See triglycerides, above.)
Remnant Lipoproteins		The more remnants, the more damage.		(See triglycerides, above.)

Source: *Environmental Nutrition*, June 2002.

The bottom line: Although the growing availability of a host of disease indicators offers valuable information, they do not supersede the established risk factors, such as elevated LDL's, low HDL's, elevated triglycerides, smoking, blood pressure, diabetes, obesity and physical inactivity. Eating well and staying active go a long way in keeping high cholesterol and heart disease at bay.

Eating Disorders: Binge Eating, Bulimia and Anorexia

Each year millions of people in the United States are affected by serious and sometimes life-threatening eating disorders. Eating disorders involve serious disturbances in eating behavior, such as extreme and unhealthy reduction of food intake or severe overeating, as well as feelings of distress or extreme concern about body shape or weight.

BINGE EATING DISORDER

Binge Eating Disorder is actually more prevalent than either Anorexia Nervosa *(anorexia)* or Bulimia Nervosa *(bulimia)* and is associated with severe obesity. A recent research study on the prevalence of eating disorders in adults living in the United States found that lifetime prevalence for Binge Eating Disorder is estimated at almost 3% of the population. In this study, to be diagnosed with Binge Eating Disorder, a person had to engage in eating binges on a regular basis for at least three months and also have attitudes or behaviors that showed a loss of control and distress. Lifetime prevalence for binge eating in general *(including both people with and without all symptoms for diagnosis)* was even higher: 4.5%. Although Binge Eating Disorder appeared to occur more often in women, the prevalence of men and women that engaged in any form of binge eating *(not necessarily at the "disorder" level)* was similar.[29]

Nearly 80% of those with Binge Eating Disorder also appeared to have some kind of psychological disorder *(including anxiety, mood, impulse-control, or substance use disorders)*, with phobias and depression occurring most frequently. People in this study reported seeking professional help for emotional and psychological concerns more than for the actual binge eating behaviors.[29] This may partially be because physicians often fail to recognize Binge Eating Disorder in their patients.[30]

People with this disorder frequently eat large amounts of food, while feeling a loss of control over their eating. This disorder is different from the binge-purge type of bulimia because people with Binge Eating Disorder usually do not purge *(by vomiting, excessive exercise, or abuse of diuretics or laxatives)* after they are done binging. People who binge on large amounts of food at one time often do so quickly and alone, to avoid discovery or embarrassment. They even eat when they are not hungry. I see many morbidly obese clients in my office who may be diagnosable, yet almost no one – at least in the beginning or maybe for many months – is willing to bring up this issue or discuss it at all. People who binge often try to hide their problem because they feel ashamed. Some say they feel disgusted, depressed or guilty after a binging episode or feel "trapped" in a downward cycle. Trying to hide the problem is common with other types of eating disorders as well.

Why Do People Binge?

- Doctors do not always know why someone has an eating disorder.
- It may be caused by the way a person's brain or body works. Researchers are looking into how brain chemicals and metabolism *(the way the body burns calories)* affect binge eating.
- People often develop the disorder as a way to cope with other problems. They may fill emotional voids in their life with food or attempt to control their lives through eating.
- Binge eating may "run" in families, possibly due to a child witnessing the behavior of a binge-eating parent over time and then modeling that behavior.

Different types of stress can lead to an eating disorder. Depression, problems with family or friends, or pressure from school or sports are examples of different types of stress. A large percentage of people with Binge Eating Disorder have a history of depression. Whether depression is a cause or effect is unclear.

From my experience, I see binging for some of my patients as a form of self-expression. "I'll do what I damn well please." It may be a form of rebellion, or an attempt to show control in one area of life while feeling helpless in other areas *(ironic, because the binging often develops into a lack of control)*.

Some use it as an escape: "While I'm eating, nothing bothers me." It may be easier to not have to deal with or think about what else is emotionally plaguing them. They may feel momentary pleasure, comfort and fulfillment through binging. Eating too much can also be a way of "getting back" at people, especially a loved one – a parent, partner, boss or sibling. "You might control some parts of my life, but you can't control how much or what I eat!"

Binging can also be a method to enlarge one's body size quickly and maintain the size that, in one's mind, "protects" him/her from social activities or unwanted advances.

Medical Risks

People who have Binge Eating Disorder and are also obese may be at risk for type 2 diabetes, high blood pressure, high cholesterol, gallbladder disease, heart disease and certain types of cancer. Self-disgust and shame related to over-eating may exacerbate psychological problems such as depression, anxiety, and substance abuse.

Treatment

Binge Eating Disorder is treatable. The earlier the diagnosis is made, the higher the percentage of success in treating this disorder. People with Binge Eating Disorder should get help from a health professional such as a psychologist and/or a psychiatrist. If you think you might have Binge Eating Disorder and your doctor does not seem familiar with or receptive to the idea, ask for a referral to a nutritionist, dietician, or psychologist. Therapy or counseling are a critical part of treatment, which should lead to better body image, an understanding why you binge and the emotions behind it, and making changes in your behaviors and possibly interpersonal relationships. Binging is commonly a form of coping. When attempting to remove that coping mechanism, it is necessary to develop other, more healthy, forms of coping to replace it.

As a nutritionist, my role involves nutritional counseling, motivation and a weight goal. By providing nutritional information and implementing a healthy diet plan, clients become aware of what, when, and how they should be eating.

Tracking eating habits with a daily diet record helps clients monitor and identify which situations are most difficult for them. Journaling helps them discover the real reasons why they binge or at least provides an outlet for expression *("venting")*. I also work with them to identify and implement substitute behaviors for their binging.

Bulimia

Bulimia Nervosa *(often called "bulimia")* is characterized by episodes of binge-eating followed by inappropriate methods of weight control. People with bulimia eat a lot of food in a short amount of time *("binges")* and then try to prevent weight gain through purging. Purging might be done by self-induced vomiting or misuse of laxatives, diet pills, or diuretics. People with bulimia may also engage in intense food restriction or strenuous, excessive exercise in order to "make up" for their binges.

During the binging episode, they experience a loss of control. Sufferers consume huge quantities of food, sometimes up to 20,000 calories at a time. The foods on which they binge tend to be "comfort foods" that are high in calories and carbohydrates. Purging is usually done in secrecy and followed by disgust and shame. It is often difficult to determine if a person is suffering from bulimia, because purging is often done in secret, and the problem is often denied. Most individuals with bulimia are of normal weight and fearful of gaining weight and feel intensely dissatisfied with their bodies.

There is no one clear cause for bulimia. Causes for bulimia may include: psychological issues *(such as stress, depression, anxiety, low-self esteem or distorted body image)*, cultural or familial influences, traumatic or stressful life events, or chemical/hormonal imbalances.

Bulimia can be very harmful to one's body in various ways. Mild health conditions may result, including: fatigue, abnormal or absent menstruation in women and irregular bowel movements. More serious health conditions can also result, including: heart failure, low blood pressure, anemia, ulcers, and dehydration.[31]

If you think you or someone you know may be experiencing symptoms of bulimia, it is extremely important that the person seek help from health professionals, including a nutritionist/dietician and a psychologist.

Anorexia

People with Anorexia Nervosa *(often called "anorexia")* have a resistance to maintain a normal body weight, due to a fear of gaining weight *(even when they are underweight)* and a distorted perception of their own body. People with this disorder see themselves as overweight even though they are often dangerously thin. The process of eating becomes an obsession, and they constantly think about their next encounter with food. They tend to pick a few foods to eat in small quantities, obsessively portion or weigh the foods, and repeatedly check their body weight. Some may exercise incessantly or use diet pills or other substances.

Anorexia is not just a problem with food or weight. It is an attempt to use food and weight to deal with emotional problems. People with this disorder may believe they would be happier and more successful if they were just thinner. They often want everything in their lives to be perfect. Obsessive eating restriction may be the only way they feel in control.

Anorexia can result in serious medical conditions, including: kidney failure, heart failure, low blood pressure, anemia, osteoporosis, and heart palpitations. Anorexia can also result in absence of menstruation in women, weak muscles and swollen joints, brittle hair and nails, constipation, bloating, fainting, lack of memory, and irritability.[31]

Treatment of anorexia is difficult because people who suffer from it often believe there is nothing wrong with them. However, if directed to counseling, they can work on becoming more aware of their unhealthy food restriction and distorted body image and the feelings that are causing their eating problems. They can then work to slowly change those behaviors and adopt a healthier lifestyle.

If you or someone you know is experiencing symptoms of anorexia, it is extremely important that the person seek help from health professionals, including a nutritionist/dietician and a psychologist. The earlier anorexia is caught and the sooner the person begins treatment, the more successful the treatment tends to be.

Resources and More Information

Eating disorders are extremely serious and more prevalent than we would like to imagine. Eating disorders affect both women and men and people of all racial/ethnic backgrounds. Sometimes just recognizing the problem is enough to prompt a change in behavior, but professional help is usually necessary and beneficial. There are numerous associations and websites available for information and help with eating disorders. Some of the websites are:

- The National Eating Disorders Association (*www.nationaleatingdisorders.org*)
- The National Women's Health Information Center: (www.*WomensHealth.gov* or *www.4woman.gov*)
- The Renfrew Center (*www.renfrewcenter.com*)
- EatingDisordersResources.org

Childhood Obesity: Super-Sizing Our Children

Is it hereditary? Is it learned? Or a little of both?! Why are so many children in America overweight? How does it begin? How can we stop it? Are we just "big" people?

Childhood obesity is now epidemic in the United States, and has attracted growing attention over the years as weight-related health problems, including type 2 diabetes, increase alongside the prevalence of overweight among children. Research through the Center for Disease Control shows that from 2003 to 2004, 17 percent of all American children and adolescents are overweight. Percentages are even slightly higher among African American and Mexican American youth. When including both children and adolescents who are overweight and also those children and adolescents who are at risk for becoming overweight, the percentage rises to 33%.[32]

Problems with Childhood Obesity

Obesity presents numerous problems for the child. In addition to increasing the risk of adulthood obesity, childhood obesity is associated with pediatric hypertension *(high blood pressure)*, type 2 diabetes, increased cholesterol levels, eating disorders, and problems with weight-bearing joints.[33] Poor self-esteem, negative self-image, depression, and withdrawal from peers have also been associated with childhood obesity.[34]

How Did This Happen?

Although there is debate regarding possible relations between genetics and obesity or biological causes, rarely is childhood obesity linked to biological causes such as thyroid or other endocrine problems. The cause is usually eating too much of the wrong foods and exercising too little. I have been frustrated by this equation for many years.

We learn specific eating habits from our parents. Many children are raised in an environment that contributes to obesity. Parents serve fatty foods, too much food, or both. Fast food could be a typical supper three or four nights a week because everyone is "too busy" to do otherwise. The old "drive-through" is the chef. Parents let their children order what they want. A typical request: "I'll have a double cheeseburger, fries and a large Coke." Your children could consume 1,300 calories for this one meal, depending on whether or not they "super-size." And not to stop there, if you get the McDonald's Triple Thick Shake, add 550 calories for the small or 1,130 calories for the large! The fat-laden path to bypass surgery is set with this quick stop... Not great for a developing child who needs certain nutrients for proper development. This food is high in cholesterol and high in fat.

We learn the good, the bad and the ugly from our parents. An overweight teen has an 80 percent chance of becoming an overweight adult. The risk of becoming obese is greatest among children with two parents that are obese. Parents are a child's model for eating and exercise behaviors. The problem is not the fast food itself, but parental supervision. We must guide our children and help them choose wisely. Go to the internet and look up the calorie, sodium and fat content of your children's favorite fast foods. Do not let your children feel like "You deserve a break today" and "Have it your way" are mantras to follow. Do not let them "super-size" their youthful bodies.

It is easier to prevent obesity than to treat it. As previously mentioned, once additional fat cells are created in your body, you will always have them. You can shrink the size of these cells, but it is still too easy to fill them back up. Obesity in children does not have to be accepted. Did you realize that fat cells primarily develop from birth to age 2 and then again from age 7 to age 12? They develop because when we eat too much *(especially as children)*, the body must create a place to store the extra calories. The common notion that "they are young and healthy, let them eat whatever they want and it won't matter" is shockingly challenged once we learn that extra fat cells developed in childhood will stay with us for life.

How big of a difference in the number of fat cells are we talking about? Obese individuals have, on average, five times the amount of fat cells as normal-weight individuals.

Exercise: What a Concept!

Yes, this is obvious...but we are just not doing it! We do not promote it, and we do not make it fun, available or required. It is true that most kids like exercise once given the opportunity *(riding a bike, throwing or kicking a ball, playing tag or other active games)*, but so much happens to reverse that desire.

Here are some verbal obstacles keeping your children from exercising: "We need ten people together to create a team activity." "I don't have the equipment." "My bike is broken." "You won't let me go to the park by myself where the other kids are." "It's too hot." "You're always too busy to throw the ball with me, Dad." "Why should I exercise? You don't do it." "I'm on the computer right now." "I've got homework/chores to do" *(a rare but effective excuse)*.

It may be true that children and adolescents' schedules are much busier than they used to be, but also look at how much time youth spend watching television or movies, playing video games, and playing on the computer. Obviously, if kids are watching TV, they are not out riding a bike or kicking a soccer ball. Physical education classes are dwindling, lost to the challenges of standardized testing. Many grade schools offer only one to two classes weekly *(or is that "weakly?")*. You can no longer count on your children getting the exercise they need at school *(sad, but true)*.

What to do? Limit "screen time" *(both television and computer)* per day. Let your child pick out his/her favorite two or three television shows that occur weekly *(for multiple children, get them to compromise)*. Put the schedule up on the refrigerator, and let them plan on watching those and only those shows, especially during the weekdays. If your children prefer computer or video games, substitute those but again, make a deal that it will be from a specific beginning time to a specific ending time each day. You will certainly encounter resistance at first, but once the child establishes consistency with the behavior, it will be much less of a battle. Ask children for their input on which and when, so they feel that they are at least partially involved in the decision. On the weekend, being more flexible can work, but only with the requirement that they do at least one active activity per day. Of course, it is not fair for you to tell your children they must change their behaviors and then have them watch you *(as a parent)* not change yours. A healthy lifestyle must be implemented at the family level.

What can you do besides limiting "screen time"? Enroll your child in a city recreational or school sports team or another active after school activity/program. Most city sports leagues are relatively inexpensive, less competitive than other leagues, and offer opportunities for all ages. Another idea is to make it a pattern to take a walk together as a family after dinner on most nights. Contact parents of other children in the neighborhood with whom your child can play with. Purchase items such as a soccer ball, basketball, Frisbee, or jump rope and have them on hand.

Education

In infancy, parent education should promote breast-feeding, delayed introduction of solid food, and tips for recognition of your child being full vs. being unhappy about something else like a dirty diaper. In early childhood, children should receive age-appropriate nutrition education, along with field trips to the grocery store to view the healthy possibilities and learn how to read labels. What are our children's favorite foods? French fries, pizza, hamburgers and ice cream. At home, children should have good parental modeling and a selection of low-fat snacks, such as fruit and granola bars, available. They should be encouraged to exercise or play sports. Television, video and computer usage should be monitored. The earlier these behaviors are introduced, the easier they are to implement *(but it is never too late)*.

The American Academy of Pediatrics *(AAP)* reports that children, on average, watch three hours of television daily and spend six and a half hours using various media *(including videos and videogames)*! Additionally, by the time the average person reaches the age of 70, he/she will have spent 7-10 years of life in front of the television! I can't imagine it! They cite research that has shown primary negative health effects on: violence and aggressive behavior, academic performance, body concept and self-esteem, sexuality, nutrition, dieting, obesity, and substance use. Apparently two thirds of all television programming contain violence, and children's shows contain the most violence of all![35] *(Convinced, yet?)*

There Is Help

Below are some suggestions for your children. For success, the entire family must be willing to institute gradual, permanent change.

- Avoid severely restricting calories from unhealthy foods. Instead, focus on permanent, gradual, lifestyle changes. For example, encouraging eating healthy snacks is more likely to elicit permanent changes than stating, "You can never have ice cream again."
- Be a good role model.
- Provide alternative, good-tasting, low-calorie snacks.
- Eat meals together, eat slowly and enjoy the mealtime.
- Don't use food as a reward or punishment.
- Don't use food as a reward or punishment *(no, this is not a typo).*
- Involve children in the meal planning and grocery shopping. If you tend to grocery shop on the same day each week, use the prior day for having a "family meal planning" meeting.
- Make eating a healthy breakfast an everyday routine. Eating breakfast starts their metabolism and feeds their brains so they will be able to concentrate in school.
- Provide routine meals that are low in fat and high in fruits and vegetables and other sources of fiber *(like whole grains).*
- Reduce your family's frequency of eating at fast food restaurants. If you do go, then learn how to make healthier choices there. See the chapter on eating out or if you use the internet, check out the fast food restaurant's website for nutritional information and healthier options. Then, you will be prepared the next time you "find yourself" there.

- Reduce sugar intake. A main contributor to obesity *(and cavities)* is sugar. Decrease the availability of soda and junk foods that are high in sugar. Encourage water as the primary beverage and make it accepted to drink only low-fat milk or water with meals.
- Encourage opportunities for physical activity. Take the kids to the park, involve your children in sports and participate in outdoor activities with them.
- Encourage your children's school to have P.E., intramural sports and recess. Get involved in the Parent-Teacher Associations to promote school cafeterias serving healthier food and removing vending machines or having only healthy choices available.
- If all else fails, prepare a healthy lunch instead of relying on the somewhat-higher-calorie school lunches. A lunch consisting of a sandwich *(use whole wheat bread and low-fat meats/cheeses)*, a piece of fruit and a granola bar does not take but only minutes to put together.
- Use the partnership program – eat right and exercise with your children. Set your goals together and you will motivate each other.

Sometimes, It's Not What Your Children Are Eating; But What's Eating Them

Many children eat in response to stress or negative emotions such as boredom, anger, sadness, anxiety or depression. Beyond the physical hazards of carrying extra weight *(which can also include high blood pressure and type 2 diabetes)*, parents need to understand the emotional problems and concerns that often underlie obesity, as well as those issues that can result from being overweight as a child. It is hard to determine which comes first, the stress causing overeating or the stress that results from being overweight.

We do know it hurts – the pain from within, the hurt from outside. "Kids say the 'darndest' things," and they are not always nice or pleasant. Bullying is a real problem in schools, on top of the stress children may place on themselves or the stress they may feel at home from family issues. Children cannot hide their pain and embarrassment. Everyone knows the pain and ostracism of being overweight. But does it have to be accepted? Some say they will grow out of it. You tell your children that they are still attractive. You know their clothes never fit right. Our advertising surreptitiously promotes obesity but rewards being thin. It is not easy, and we cannot just turn our heads and deny that overweight children have not or are not experiencing some kind of psychological turmoil from being overweight.

When was the last time your child came home crying because of insults at school? When did your child last tell you she was the last person chosen for the team? Why didn't your 12 year-old take off his shirt at the beach?

Consider the following when dealing with your overweight/obese child and their emotions:

- Your child may have turned to food to camouflage feelings and emotions.
- They need your encouragement, love and support. You must tell them and not expect them to "know" that you love and support them.
- Positive parental attention of any type helps create positive self-esteem.
- Become alert to your child's experiencing stresses at school or with peers. Gently encourage them to tell you when something is bothering them. Tell them that you care about them and that you will listen.
- Talk with your child about experiencing teasing at school and positive ways to respond.
- Realize that emotional eating of junk food provides temporary emotional "comfort."
- Parents need to focus on health, not appearance.
- Encourage and participate with your children in physical activity.
- Help them by getting them involved with meal planning, give them choices *(such as letting them choose which vegetable they want from the store)*.
- Tell your child that you are going to make changes together *(and then do!)*, because you both want to be healthy.
- Always remind them that you care!

Case Histories

"There are eight million stories in the naked city," to borrow a line from an old TV detective show, yet too many of these stories are failures. The successes are those who change their habits and behaviors and have the awareness of what they can do for themselves.

The following are a few select stories of some of my clients who have succeeded against all odds. As discussed earlier, my opinion is that successful weight has occurred when someone loses weight *(no matter how much)* and then manages to keep that weight off. Most people – as we all know – gain it back, because they have not really changed those habits and behaviors that have caused them to become overweight in the first place.

These people highlighted in the case histories below have succeeded. I am proud of them, but most importantly, they are incredibly proud of themselves. I believe that you will be motivated and inspired by reading about their struggles and ultimate successes...I certainly am.

These names are fictional, but the people and their stories are fact.

Tanisha, What Success!

Tanisha was a 36 year-old African American woman, with two young teenage boys and no job. She weighed 434 pounds, had sleep apnea and high blood pressure.

When a local government agency that pays for medical and

vocational rehabilitation referred her to me, she could barely walk and came to my office half asleep. With my usual information form and subsequent one-on-one questioning, I learned:

She ate one meal a day: supper. It usually consisted of a high-fat meat, almost no starches, and no veggie *(said she couldn't afford them)*. She reported that her kids were constantly "acting up,"almost out of her control. She had no transportation other than the bus. The first day in my office, she almost fell asleep on my desk *(sleep apnea will do that to you)*.

I said to her, "I realize all the weight loss battles you have been through in your life. Yet, you must know that, in my opinion, your only chance of succeeding now is water walking." She didn't say a word. I went on. "Go to Myers Park Pool *(a local city pool that is heated in the winter)* five days a week, get into the pool in chest-high water, and walk around for 20 minutes daily. You will lose weight. Your knees won't hurt you; your feet will support you; your back will be OK. Give it a chance. If you don't try this, there is no sense in coming back here, no matter how much I would like to help you."

I can never tell a book by its cover. In her first follow-up session, Tanisha told me she had been to the pool three times that week and had begun writing down her meals, using my daily food diary. Her attitude had changed from disillusionment to feeling motivated. Every week she improved. She saw a small, dim light in the darkness and carefully followed it.

Fast forward to one year later: Tanisha had lost 115 pounds *(from 434 pounds to 319 pounds!)* through water walking, recording her meals, changing her diet, and not intentionally skipping any meals. By now, her attitude had really changed. The government rehabilitation program paid for her sessions, the pool entry fees, and the bus fare. They also trained her in a vocation. She had a job, she had hope, and she had some real, tangible evidence of success...and all this continued to motivate her.

The second year, she was able to walk on land and no longer needed to go to the pool, which had become inconvenient because of her new job. She lost 75 more pounds *(now down to 244!)*. At the end of her third year, the last year I counseled her, she had lost A TOTAL OF 234 POUNDS!

One day, she came into my office, dressed to the nines. She looked terrific and was only 200 pounds *(recall: she was originally 434 pounds)*. What a metamorphosis! Attitude, awareness, habits, behavior, routine...the changes were solid and omnipresent. The last time I saw her was seven years later, and she had still kept off her weight. She was amazing, and the change in her life was amazing. Tanisha, what a success!

Steve, a Gastric Bypass Failure

Steve weighed 400 pounds in high school. At only 19 years of age, he had gastric bypass surgery. He lost 85 pounds. Finally, after this major surgical procedure, he was seemingly on the road to weight-loss success. He then discovered that, despite the surgical procedure making his stomach smaller, he could eat food in very small quantities, but often. Herein lies the problem! The only date he had ever had in his young life was a large pizza on a Saturday night. He would eat it a little at a time throughout the evening, until he went to bed, sometimes at 3:00 in the morning.

When he was 30 years old, he showed up at my office. Steve weighed 381 pounds, still morbidly obese even after having had the gastric bypass surgery. He had *(like most people)* been looking for the "quick fix," the easiest possible way to lose weight. By this point in his life, he had already been down that road, and the "quick-fix" clearly hadn't worked for him. So, when we first discussed behaviors and strategies, he was ready...very ready...to finally do something different.

Instead of: skipping breakfast, having a large lunch, grazing at supper and all-night binging, he began his new routine. His "quest" for a healthy life had begun. He even began exercising by walking. Embarrassed by his size, he would walk at 5 a.m. in his neighborhood, when no one was outside.

The Saturday night "date pizza" became a smaller version, and eventually he began going out to dinner with friends, using his new portion control techniques when choosing meals. Eventually, he had a date. The first normal date of his life became a steady girlfriend for about a year. By this time, he was down from 381 pounds to 256 pounds! At 6'1" tall, he was looking pretty good. He had gained a lot of self-confidence and even became open to sharing both his challenges and successes with others. Eventually, he stopped losing weight and backed off his frequency of exercising, but continued to use the "portion control habits" that have kept his weight down. Together, we were able to do what a surgical procedure couldn't! Alright, Steve!

Melanie, My Poster Child

Melanie showed up one day with a "walker", one of those metal support frames that you place in front of you as you walk forward. This is unusual – I thought to myself – a 37 year-old woman using a walker.

It turned out that five years earlier, she had been in a terrible car accident. She had metal rods in her back and had lost the portion of her leg below the knee. She weighed 320 pounds and had one leg. Her life was challenging, to say the least. Obviously, whatever weight she could lose would greatly improve her mobility.

I showed her how, and she did the rest. I told her that you have to say to yourself, "Enough is enough. I do not want to be this person anymore." Because of her accident and her size, Melanie's ability to move had been greatly reduced. The walker or even a wheelchair could be her future.

Slow-moving, careful steps were all she could do. But she compensated for her inability to exercise by cutting back on portions, eating the right foods, and timing her meals. Through establishing a routine of healthy eating and portion-control, she achieved success. She obviously realized the smaller and lighter her body was, the better her mobility would be, and this motivated her to put my suggestions into action.

Again, I can never tell a book by its cover. One year later, she had lost 118 pounds! She was down from 320 to 202 pounds! One leg, and yet, she was so successful! Once she lost 50 pounds, her surgeon had to fit her for a smaller artificial leg!

Melanie's goal was to weigh 150 pounds *(from the original 320 lbs)*. She is on her way. She is on *"The Path"* and is changing her habits, behavior, lifestyle and attitude. She is a source of motivation for all.

If she can do it, you can do it.

Betty, Heavy and Hypoglycemic

I'm standing in the check-out line at a local grocery store. The woman in front of me, writing a check for the cashier, turns to me and proclaims, "You're Dr. Kaye! You probably don't remember me, but you saved my life!"

Wow! I looked around and realized that yes, she was talking to me. I didn't recognize her, but I quickly filtered through my memory to recall if I ever saved a drowning person or performed some other impressive life-saving event. Hmm, no.... She must be talking about my nutritional practice.

She went on to tell me how 8 or 10 years earlier, she had been 75 pounds overweight, depressed and even suicidal. She came to me in desperation to lose weight. During my initial evaluation, I had learned: Betty had experienced symptoms that which were at least partially caused by the "highs and lows" of her blood sugar. She not only did not have any routine when it came to meals, but she also had a history of both diabetes and hypoglycemia in her family.

Betty had been diagnosed with Bipolar Disorder *(previously known as Manic-Depressive Disorder)*, put on psychiatric medication, and then left alone by her counselor. During our initial discussion, I realized that her highs and lows could be partially self-created, due to lack of eating routine and timing of her meals. When her blood sugar dropped, she became lethargic and emotionally down. So then, she ate, but often too late for her blood sugar to recover. Besides experiencing these lows, when she finally ate, her metabolism "backed up," holding on to whatever the body was ingesting and storing it *(causing weight gain)*.

We worked with her counselor to get her into a regular eating routine and gradually decrease her medication. In two or three months, she no longer needed the medication! In about a year's time, she had lost 50 pounds. She met her goal-weight within the following year. More importantly, by eating on a routine schedule, she learned how to control her blood sugar, which greatly helped to control her mood swings *(highs and lows)*. Since the end of that first year, I had not seen her until I saw her in the grocery store that day, many years later. Her success had been terrific, lasting, and obviously life-altering. She was now in control of her life in many positive ways that she did not think were even possible before. The consequences of changing her lifestyle had been so powerful that she had felt her life had been "saved."

Pam, Everything is Possible!
(real name, by permission)

It's wonderful to see the hippie mentality still exists, thrives and can be successful. I have learned I can never tell a book by its cover. When Pam came to me she weighed 351 pounds. We went through my whole program and she began a process of change. Whatever changed mentally – her attitude about herself, her goals, her self-esteem – caused an enormous change externally. She was ready no to be a grossly overweight person anymore. Getting into a routine of living daily enabled Pam to change most, if not all, of the habits that have caused her weight gain. It is all about attitude, the "can-do" attitude. She began keeping a daily diet record of her food intake, before eating and continues to walk daily for 30 to 40 minutes. In a year, from November 13, 2002 until November 13, 2003, she lost 144 pounds. Currently, she weighs 170 pounds even after experiencing "the holidays" – Thanksgiving through New Year's – without gaining any weight. Don't think she was perfect during the holidays though she remained steadfast with walking, which in the long run will help maintain her weight. Stay tuned folks. Pam could be the poster child. Mover over Jared *(Subway)*! Go Pam!

267

Testimonials

You have just read the Case Histories of a few of my client "success stories." Each person had their own major life challenges, and each was able to overcome those challenges in order to achieve their goals of losing weight and adopting a healthier lifestyle. Those stories were from my perspective. However, hearing first-hand is often even more powerful. A few of my clients were open and comfortable enough to share their own experience with weight loss. I thank them sincerely and hope that reading someone else's account will help you to feel that you can achieve these goals as well.

From: Pam

Hi. My name is Pam and by following Dr. Kaye's program, I have achieved goals that I hadn't dreamed were possible. I have confidence in myself again. I'm proud of what I have done. It amazes me daily. Seeing positive results has fortified my faith beyond my dreams. Staying steadfast in the course Dr. Kaye has chartered for me, I have become a new person ... or rather, I've become me!

Fourteen months ago, I was sad, very ill health. I had put myself in a new situation, out of desperation, and all of a sudden, serious thing started happening to my health. Sleep apnea was the primary diagnosis that referred me to Dr. Kaye. The worst event was falling asleep behind the wheel of a running car. Then there were the embarrassing moments like falling asleep when the "Big Boss: attempted to engage me in conversation. Once, in the early stages of a staff meeting, I awoke with

Pam

Before

After

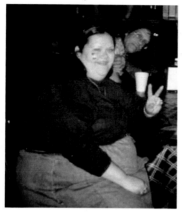

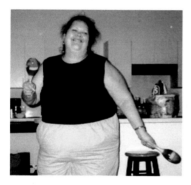

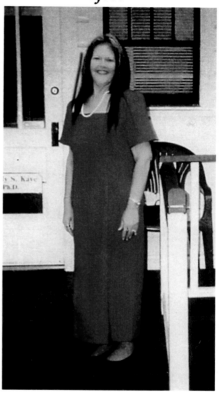

a start – realizing I had fallen asleep yet again. There were about ten more "things" on my list, but the sleep apnea – interruption of sleep because physical problems, such as narrow air passageway or, excess tissue inside the throat – was directly related to obesity. Those layers upon layers of jelly rolls on my chest, breasts, throat and neck were suffocating me every night.

Only two possible remedies were available to me. One was to have reconstructive surgery on my face to either re size my sinus cavities, nasal passages and or possibly throat diameter. The other was to get my weight into a normal range something I have maybe only been twice in my adult life.

I received a call from my primary-care physician's office informing me of a referral to Dr. Kaye, someone who I knew from my junior and senior years at Florida State University. He had been in the doctoral program but had an office in the College of Hotel and Restaurant Administration. His office was next to one of my "coolest" college professors, and he had been asked to give a lecture to one of my afternoon classes because tat professor had a family emergency. I knew he was a great motivator and the he might be able to help me.

I was scared and embarrassed of what I had become. And now I had to face someone who had gone forward, who had done so well, and here I was just an out-right mess.

Dr. Kaye gave me his plan along with a bonus of some much needed counseling. He taught Me: There are no problems we cannot solve with determination. Each of us has it in us. You can be what you want when you grow up!

It's a good thing I'm not there yet!

Kindest Regards
Pam

P.S. Just so you'd know, as of this writing, I have decided to go back to college and pursue advanced education in nutrition and find some opportunities involving community education with an emphasis in childhood obesity. This dream will take on some more refinement as time passes, but I will keep telling myself, "I know I Can. I know I can, I will."

From: Incredible Mel
(okay, I put in the "incredible" part)

I am very honored to be a part of Dr. Freddy Kaye's book. I met Dr. Kaye about a year and a half ago. Thank God!

In 1997, I was horribly injured in a car accident. My back was fused and my right leg was amputated. For six years, I had been in and out of hospitals and rehabilitation centers. I had numerous surgeries, and had to fight hard to ward off terrible infections.

During those years, my weight fluctuated up and down and depression was definitely a factor. Dr. Kaye had a great impact on my life. First, he made me aware of what I was eating by giving me booklets to record was I was going to have for breakfast, lunch and dinner. He introduced me to new foods and a new style of eating. I could hear his voice telling me: "DON'T MAKE FOOD SO IMPORTANT!"

Whenever I faced a food challenge, he would say to me: "Stay focused. What do you really want?" I wanted to be able to walk and start working again. I wanted my lifestyle to change. My grandfather told me I could do anything I wanted to do. Dr. Kaye reinforced his wisdom. Those words stand true in any aspect of life.

Now, I have lost more than 100 pounds. I'm walking well on my prosthetic and have returned to work as a hair dresser. Dr. Kaye, with his counseling and encouragement, played a big part in helping me reach my goals.

> *Thank you so much, Dr. Kaye.*
> *Melanie McClain*

Note: Melanie was 275 pounds at 37 years old when she began my program. As of this writing, she weighed 159 pounds.

From: Pastor Vance

For many years, I over-indulged, lived in sedentary comfort, assumed I was genetically "big-boned", found countless excuses for my weight, and occasionally tried a fad diet. One day, I realized that I was robbing myself of "quality of life" in the short run and "quantity of life" in the long run.

I was on the verge of diabetes and heart disease and in a state of extreme obesity and fatigue. My physician gave me two alternatives: undergo gastric bypass surgery or learn some accountability by beginning a regimen with a nutritionist. Being afraid of knives and pain, I chose the nutritionist, Dr. Freddy Kaye.

Though radical lifestyle change is never easy, Dr. Kaye introduced me to a set of values that has made an amazing difference in the quality of my life. After eight months, I have lost 80 pounds, with approximately 40 pounds to go. I've learned to make better food choices, practice portion control, have a dietary plan, and most importantly, I've developed a routine to live by. I now consciously choose things that will provide long-term gratification - health, energy, better self-image - instead of comforting myself with the immediate gratification of high-cost, low-yield food.

Dr. Kaye's plan is not a "diet" in the common use of the word. It isn't a program that one uses to drop a few pounds and then return to former habits and former weight gain. This is a practical, health-centered, historically and universally-based nutritional plan for eating right and living well.

Thank you, Dr. Kaye, for giving me back my life and for teaching me a better way to eat and live.

Dr. Vance C. Rains

Pastor/Director
Florida State University
Wesley Foundation

Note: *1 1/2 years after going on the program, Pastor Vance is now down to 206 pounds, from 330 pounds.*

From: Laura, the ER Nurse

When I went to Dr. Freddy Kaye's office 14 months ago, I weighed 378 1/2 pounds. I was desperate and had decided to have gastric bypass surgery. It was my last resort. I had arthritis and knee problems and was almost immobile, not a good thing for an emergency room nurse. I feared I would soon be unable to walk.

However, before it would approve the surgery, my insurance plan required that I participate in a weight-management program for a year. I had done these types of programs unsuccessfully for years and told them that unless they sent me to the right person, it would be futile for me to just go through the motions.

Dr. Kaye was the right person. He was different – he has a kind of 60's mentality and genuinely listened to what I had to say. I cried, but he was straight with me. He said he would give it his best shot but said I would have to give it my best shot also.

We came up with a food plan that was convenient and that had foods that I enjoyed. He also recommended that I start exercising but, at my size, that was hard to consider. I walked at work but only for short periods at a time. But he was encouraging, and I walked out of his office with hope.

By my next visit, which was after the holidays, I had lost nine pounds. The following visit was disappointing. I had lost less than a pound.

Freddy said part of my problem was that my erratic work schedule didn't allow me to establish a routine. That was frustrating to me. I couldn't quit my job. I loved it.

When I left his office, my first thought was to head straight to Burger King for a Double Whopper with Cheese. But I knew I wouldn't be hurting him, I'd be hurting me. I won that battle and decided to talk with my boss to see if we could adjust my schedule. Knowing my situation, he agreed.

Next, I had to learn how to change my eating habits. It wasn't easy. I couldn't go from eating 5,000 to 6,000 calories a day to 1,000 – even dropping to 1,500 was hard.

Sometimes I'd get so hungry I couldn't stop eating, but gradually that changed. I started eating small meals more frequently to keep by blood sugar from dropping. It also helped keep that intense hunger from taking over. I started counting calories. I learned to enjoy a low-fat turkey sandwich with a tablespoon of mayonnaise. Working under my doctor's care, I used diet pills to get me through the transition.

I knew there was some controversy about this method but, to me, it was the lesser of two evils. I got through it, gave up the pills and began losing weight. After failing at every diet under the sun for 27 years, I had found one that worked!

I finally opened some walking tapes I had ordered months before. The first one was for a mile walk, but I could only make it a half mile at first. It hurt, both in my back and knees, but I kept going. Freddy was right, it became part of my routine.

Gradually, with the help of Motrin, I worked through the pain. Every day, I could go further, and I now walk 45 minutes each day, going about three miles. I don't do it because I enjoy it – I still count the minutes till it's over – but because I can now cross my legs and no longer have to order my clothes from magazines. I also do it out of fear that if I stop, I won't start again and will face a lifetime of immobility.

So far, I've lost 130 pounds and feel more physically and emotionally healthy than I ever have. I have my ups and downs. I recently had a "bad" month in which I probably had a little too much to drink. I also went through a period of depression and missed walking for three days. But with Freddy's encouragement, I dragged myself out of it. He's taught me that no matter how strong you are, there are times that you will fail. You just have to keep trying.

What I learned from him is that it's necessary to find a plan that fits you. Exercise, watch what goes in your mouth, and keep it easy and convenient.

Thank you, Dr. Freddy Kaye. I don't know why it worked this time, but I know you have been an inspiration and a wealth of knowledge. You know I haven't always agreed with you – it has taken me time to learn or unlearn certain behaviors. But you are always understanding and full of ideas to help me with my problem areas concerning food. You believe in what you do, and thank you for believing in me.

Laura

From: **Alan**

At age 38 and closing in on my 20th wedding anniversary, I weighed close to 360 pounds. On my wedding day, I had weighed 165 pounds and every anniversary thereafter the scales went up. I realized I couldn't keep putting on weight year after year and decided to do something about it. Over the next two years, my weight "yo-yoed" down to about 290 pounds and then right back up to 325. After seeing pictures of myself from my son's high school graduation, I knew I needed help. I went to my physician, expecting to get some kind of written diet plan or to be told I needed bypass surgery. What I got was a referral to Dr. Freddy Kaye.

On my initial visit, Dr. Kaye explained his program. It sounded like the same old song – eat less, exercise more. But, instead of handing me a pre-printed menu plan or a gimmick system to trade-off foods, he talked to me about my personal challenges and gave me simple alternatives to what I had been doing.

I had wanted to know how to eat healthy, and Dr. Kaye's program taught me just that. Knowing why certain foods were good for me motivated me to make better, healthier choices. I thought I would have to buy a lot of specialty foods to survive while losing weight, but that wasn't the case. I just had to learn to buy healthier foods.

When I started Dr. Kaye's program, I weighed 323 pounds and could barely walk two miles without giving out. A year later, after eating healthier food and exercising regularly, I'm 120 pounds lighter and do a range of activities I couldn't do before I started with Dr. Kaye – jog, water ski, bicycle and enjoy amusement parks.

My cholesterol levels and blood pressure have improved tremendously. All of these things have added to my life but most importantly, these changes have given me a chance for a longer life to spend with my family.

Alan Kirkland

Ruth

Before

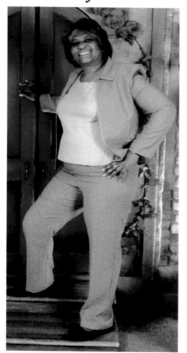

After

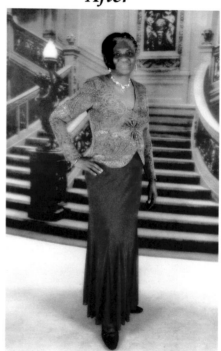

Jon

Before   *After*

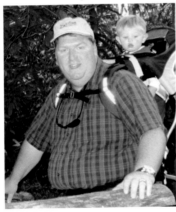

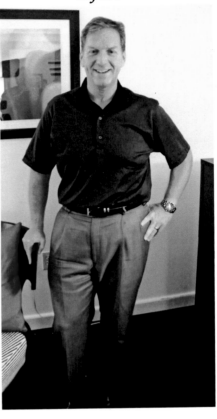

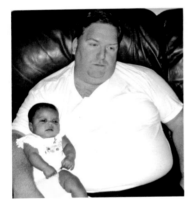

Keeping "It" Off, Staying On The Program

Long-term weight loss escapes most of us. The concept of losing weight and successfully keeping it off is foreign to our thinking *(or at least to our experience)*. I have been counseling overweight and obese people for 26 years. Invariably, the thought of actually having to change the lifestyle and habits that caused the weight gain in the first place is no easy task.

Yet, think about it, please. You have to alter, change, modify whatever you have been doing or thinking which has resulted in your becoming overweight or obese. This book and the program within it have been designed to show you exactly how to accomplish this monumental and rare task. You can do it! Just follow my suggestions: discipline, routine, portion control, educated choices, exercise, honesty, delayed gratification, and not blaming others or the situation for your weight problems. Take charge! If you have the desire to not be this overweight/obese person anymore, then do it and do it daily. When you've blown it *(it will happen)*, pick yourself up and get right back on *The Path*, each and every time. You can do it. Each new meal is an opportunity to put yourself right back on track.

Pretty soon, by learning how to take charge and knowing how to get back on the program, you won't be "blowing it" as often. It is your body and your life. You are in control.

I have seen it work for years, for many individuals who have battled their weight much of their adult and even childhood lives. If my program didn't work, I couldn't have possibly made a living at helping people succeed at something they normally have repeatedly failed in.

The only way you will lose weight and keep "It" off is by permanently changing your thinking, attitude, awareness, habits and behaviors, which will result in:

- Automatically thinking and planning ahead for each meal and food-related situation.
- Locking in a routine time or schedule to exercise *(walk)* regularly, five days per week minimum.
- Getting use to lesser amounts of food, focusing on: portions, portions, portions.
- Believing that each day can be a new beginning.
- Not beating yourself up for "blowing it." Realizing that you will sometimes make mistakes and that that's okay.
- Learning from your mistakes and failures *(once you've been burned at the stove why touch it again?)*

Honestly, I believe I said it before Nike:
"Just Do It" ... and Do It, and Do It, and Keep on Doing It!

IF YOU SAY "I CAN" THEN YOU WILL.

All the Best,
Freddy Kaye

References

1) Centers for Disease Control and Prevention *(CDC)*. (2008, March 6). Nutrition for everyone: Protein. Retrieved March 30, 2008, from http://www.cdc.gov/nccdphp/dnpa/nutrition/nutrition_for_everyone/basics/protein.htm#How%20much%20protein

2) Brownell, K.D. *(2000). The LEARN program for weight management.* Dallas, TX: American Health Publishing Company.

3) National Center for Health Statistics. *(2006).* Chartbook on trends in the health of Americans, 2006. Hyattsville, MD: Public Health Service.

4) Pennington, J.A.T. *(1989). Food values of portions commonly used (15th ed.).* New York, NY: Harper Collins.

5) Denke, M.A., & Grundy, S.M. *(1991).* Effects of fats high in stearic acid on lipid and lipoprotein concentrations in men. *The American Journal of Clinical Nutrition, 54,* 1036-1040. Retrieved January 27, 2007 from http://www.ajcn.org/cgi/content/abstract/54/6/1036

6) United States Department of Agriculture. *(2002).* Agriculture fact book, 2001-2002. Washington, D. C.: United States Department of Agriculture.

7) International Diabetes Foundation. *(2007).* Diabetes prevalence. Retrieved July 16, 2007, from http://www.idf.org/home/index.cfm?node=264

8) International Diabetes Foundation. *(2007).* Summary of IDF consensus on the prevention of type 2 diabetes: High-risk approach. Retrieved July 16, 2007, from http://www.idf.org/home/index.cfm?unode=C89A2F06-AOF1-487AC-91AA38AC94DEFEB4

9) Cho, F., Chen, W.Y., Hunter, D.J., Stampfer, M.J., Colditz, G.A., Hankinson, S.E., & Willett, W.C. *(2006).* Red meat intake and risk of breast cancer among premenopausal women. *Archives of Internal Medicine, 166,* 2253-2259.

10) Ziegler, R. G., Hoover, R. N., Pike, M.C., Heldesheim, A., Nomura, A. M., West, D.W., Wu-Williams, A.H., et al. *(1993).* Migration patterns and breast cancer risk in Asian-American women. *Journal of the National Cancer Institute, 85,* 1819-1827.

11) Blackburn, G.L., Copeland, T., Khaodhiar, L., & Buckley, R.B. *(2003).* Diet and breast cancer. *Journal of Women's Health, 12,* 183-192.

12) Chan, J. M., Gan, P.H., & Giovannucci, E.L. *(2005)*. Role of diet in prostate cancer development and progression. *Journal of Clinical Ontology, 23,* 8152-8160.

13) Martínez, M.E. *(2005)*. Primary prevention of colorectal cancer: Lifestyle, nutrition, exercise. *Recent Results of Cancer Research, 166,* 177-211.

14) Burkitt, D.P. *(1971)*. Epidemiology of cancer of the colon and rectum. *Cancer, 28,* 3-13.

15) Schatzkin, A. Lanza, E., Freedman, L.S., Tangrea, J., Cooper, M.R., Marshall, J.R., Murphy, P.A., et al. *(1996)*. The polyp prevention trial 1: Rational, design, recruitment, and baseline participant characteristics. *Cancer Epidemiology, Biomarkers, & Preventions, 5,* 375-383.

16) Ornish, D., Scherwitz, L. W., Billings, J.H., Gould, K.L., Merri, T.A., Sparler, S., Armstrong, W.T., et al. *(1998)*. Intensive lifestyle changes for reversal of coronary heart disease. *Journal of the American Medical Association, k280,* 2001-2007.

17) American Obesity Association. *(2005, May 2)*. Health effects of obesity. Retrieved July 14, 2007, from http://obesity1.tempdomainname.com/subs/fastfacts/Health_Effects.shtml

18) American Obesity Association. *(2005, May 2)*. AOA fact sheets: Obesity in minority populations. Retrieved July 16, 2007, from http://obesity1.tempdomainname.com/subs/fastfacts/Obesity_Minority_Pop.shtml

19) Sherman, H.C. *(1920)*. Calcium requirement in man. *Journal of Biological Chemistry, 44,* 21-27.

20) Hegsted, D.M. *(1986)*. Calcium and osteoporosis. *Journal of Nutrition, 116,* 2316-2319.

21) Robertson, W. G., Heyburn, P.J., Peacock, M., Hanes, F.A., & Swaminathan, R. *(1979)*. The effect of high animal protein intake on the risk of calcium stone-formation in the urinary tract. *Clinical Science, 57,* 285-288.

22) Huffington, A. *(2002, Feb 14)*. Drugs in our food = national security? Retrieved March 2, 2007 from http://www.alternet.org/story/12419/

23) Hellmich, N. Weighing the cost: Is being fat an illness that should be covered by insurance? USA TODAY. *(21 January 2002)*: 1D.

24) United States Department of Agriculture: National Agriculture Library. *(2007, August 4)*. Dietary reference intakes: Macronutrients. Retrieved September 15, 2007, from http:// www.iom.edu/Object.File/Master /7/300/Webtabemacro.pgf

25) Oldways Preservation Trust: Whole Grains Council. *(2007)*. Whole grains 101. Retrieved October 1, 2007, from http://www.wholegrains council.org/wholegraines-101

26) Burkitt, D.P. *Eat Right - To Stay Healthy and Enjoy Life More : How Simple Diet Changes Can Prevent Many Common Diseases.* New York: Arco Publishing, 1979.

27) United States Environmental Protection Agency. *(2004).* What you need to know about mercury in fish and shellfish. Retrieved November 7, 2007, from http://www.epa.gov/waterscience/ fish advice/advice.html#tuna

28) Antinoro, L. *(2002).* Leaving cholesterol in the dust: New ways to predict heart disease. *Environmental Nutrition, 25,* 1-4. Retrieved September 17, 2007, from the EBSCOhost database.

29) Hudson, J. L., Hiripi, E., Pope, H.G., & Kessler, R.C. *(2007).* The prevalence and correlates of eating disorders in the National Comorbidity Survey of Replication. *Biological Psychiatry, 61,* 348-358.

30) Johnson, J.G., Spitzer, R.L., & Williams, J.B. *(2001).* Health problems, impairment and illnesses associated with bulimia nervosa and binge eating disorder among primary care and obstetric gynecology patients. *Psychological Medicine, 31,* 1455-1466.

31) National Women's Health Information Center: United States Department of Health and Human Services. *(2007).* Eating disorders. Retrieved October 30, 2007, from http://www.4woman.gov/bodyimage/eatingdisorders/

32) National Center for Health Statistics: Centers for Disease Control and Prevention *(2007, November 6).* NCHS 2004 fact sheet: Obesity still a major problem, new data show. Retrieved November 2, 2007, from http://www.cdc.gov/ nchs/pressroom/06facts/obesity03_04.htm

33) The Trust of America's Health. *(2006).* F as in fat: How obesity policies are failing in America, 2006. Retrieved October 29, 2007, from http://wwwhealthyamerians.org/reports/obesity2006/

34) American Obesity Association. *(2002).* Childhood obesity. Retrieved October 20, 2007, from http://obesity1.tempdomainname.com/subs/childhood/ healthrisks.shtml

35) American Academy of Pediatrics. *(2001).* Children, adolescents, and television. *Pediatrics, 107(2).*

About the Author

DR. FREDDY KAYE'S educational background and extensive work experience have well provided him with the knowledge, strategies, and motivational skills necessary to help his clients adopt a healthier lifestyle. ■ For 30 years as a Clinical Nutritionist, Dr. Kaye has maintained a busy private practice, counseling patients *(adults, youth, couples, and families)* in nutrition, weight loss, weight management, and diet-related diseases such as heart disease and diabetes. B.A fromTulane University. ■ Dr. Kaye received a Master of Science in Nutrition and Food Science in 1977 from Florida State University. In 1980, he completed his PhD in Adult Education from Florida State University, specializing in Nutrition Education. ■ Dr. Kaye's research on weight control and behavior modification was published in 1982 in *The American Journal of Clinical Nutrition*. For 20 years, Dr. Kaye has been on the faculty of the Family Practice Residency Program of Tallahassee Memorial Regional Medical Center, teaching nutrition and diet therapy to physicians-in-training. He also serves as an Adjunct Professor at Florida A&M University. ■ Dr. Kaye is an active public speaker and has presented to numerous health and professional organizations. ■ Dr. Kaye has also appeared on television talk shows, written a weekly health column in *The Tallahassee Democrat*, and has been interviewed on CNN.